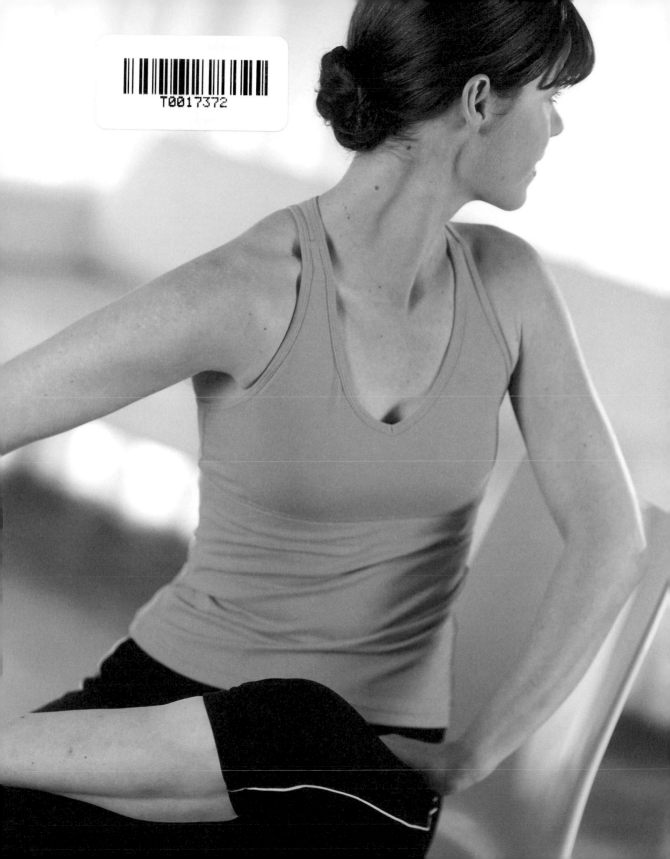

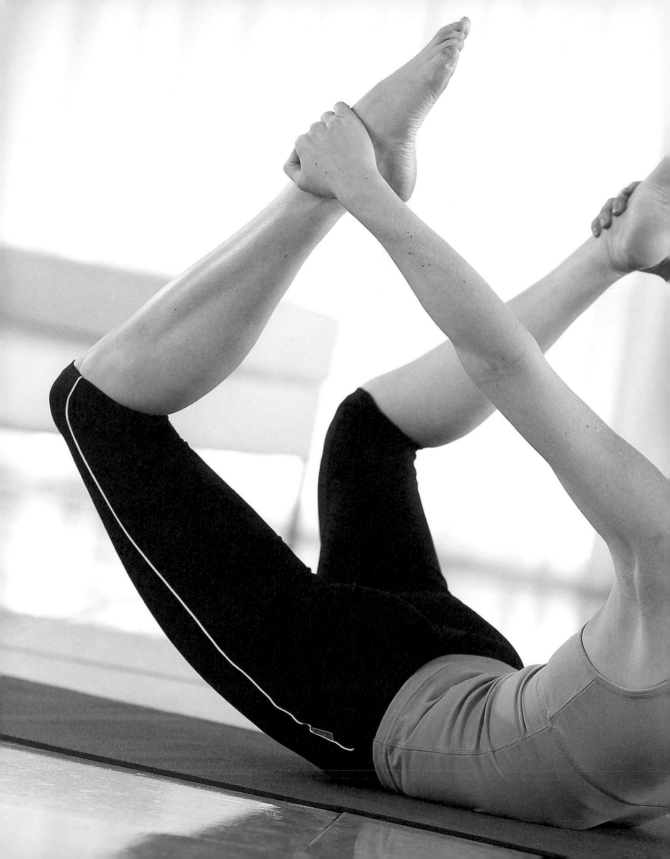

15 MINUTE
STRETCH

Suzanne Martin P.T., D.P.T.

HEALTH WARNING

All participants in fitness activities must assume the responsibility for their own actions and safety. If you have any health problems or medical conditions, consult with your physician before undertaking any of the activities in this book. The information contained in this book cannot replace sound judgment and good decision making, which can help reduce risk of injury. Neither the author nor the publisher shall be liable or responsible for any loss or damage allegedly arising from any information or suggestion in this book.

CONTENTS

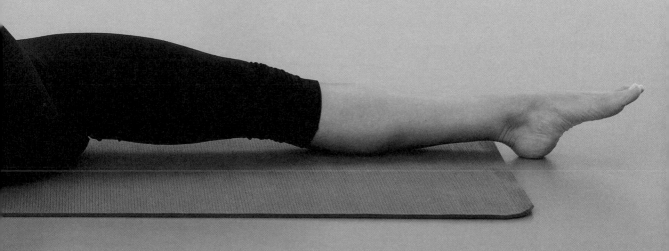

PREFACE

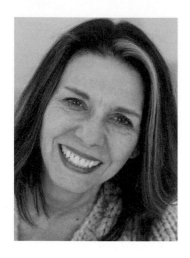

Here it is! Thanks to all of you who enjoyed my first stretching book, and especially to all of you who contacted me to request more stretching and succeeded in exerting your influence in spurring the production of this book. Here are four themes with stretches that have been a part of my regimen for years. A special welcome to those of you new to stretching. May you become a lifelong convert!

Stretching is an integral part of body maintenance, as essential as brushing your teeth. Please don't be misled into thinking of it as a competitive sport, where more is better. This is not the case. Stretching is for everyone, male or female, naturally flexible or uncomfortably stiff. Correct stretching changes how your whole body looks, as well as providing pain relief and reducing stress.

Keep your mind open. Some of the instructions given may seem prescriptive, but that is because the effectiveness of the stretches lies in the setup. Many people spend years in the gym, yet never seem to gain results. They don't pay attention to their setup.

Look hard at the pictures and tips. The explanations will help you organize the exercise concepts in your mind, which will help you organize the efforts in your body to gain the greatest effect. This may take time, so be patient.

The stretches will reveal where your body needs help. Observe and compare one side of your body to the other. Can you feel both sides "organizing themselves" into the movement or position? Is any body part talking to you? Please remember that our supple models are only demonstrators. Follow the instructions, mimic the basic shapes, and understand the cues. Then take the movements further. Internalize them until you can feel every bone inside your body. Learn to compare the way your body stretches today to the way it stretched yesterday. Don't compare it with the model's body.

Learn to see your body as it is. The famous composer Stravinsky once said that once he knew his limitations, then he could become creative. Until we see our bodies as they really are, and respect their individuality, we won't bring about change.

Take the challenge. Construct a new, improved you. These simple exercises hold a key to your body's potential. Permanent change happens one little increment at a time. Each 15-minute segment will bring you closer to a more wonderful you. Enjoy.

Dr. Suzanne Martin

HOW TO USE THIS BOOK

Stretch toward a new you! Each of the four programs in this book uses stretching to develop different aspects of your body. Think of those aspects like the facets of a diamond, honed with precision by the diamond cutter so that each one sparkles and makes a glorious whole.

This book shows you how to transform your body—and your life—through stretching. Each stretch stands by itself, but when done in sequence, there is a powerful cumulative effect. To start, read the introduction to each program to get an idea of its theme. Next, try the program for yourself, then read the FAQs pages and annotations, and study the "feel-it-here" outlines on the exercise pages to learn more and make the moves your own.

Certain stretches will be harder for some people than for others, depending on your experience and body type. Remember, there's always an easier way, so use the modifications given in the FAQs and on pp100–101. Remember, too, that you need to do a variety of movements in many different planes in order to identify weak links in your body.

There's no such thing as an easy exercise. Any exercise or stretch, however simple it may seem, brings greater benefits the more mindfully you do it.

The video available at www.dk.com/15-minute-stretch is designed to be used with the book if you want to reinforce the exercises. As you watch the video, page references to the book flash up on screen. Refer to these for more detailed instruction.

THE SUMMARIES
The summaries at the end of each sequence show you each stretch sequence as a whole. Once you've watched the video, and examined the modifications and tips for each exercise, the summary will help reinforce the sense of the sequence and give you a quick at-a-glance reference. More importantly, when

working without the video, you can also use the summary to prolong a stretch and linger from stretch to stretch, embellishing and savoring each.

SAFETY ISSUES
Be sure to get clearance from your doctor or healthcare provider before you begin any new exercise program. The advice and exercises in this book are not intended to be a substitute for individual medical help.

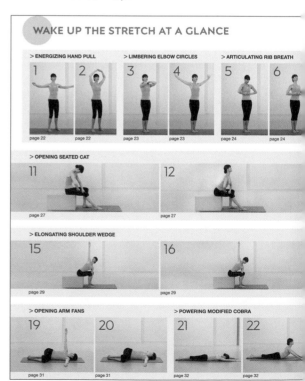

WAKE UP THE STRETCH AT A GLANCE

> ENERGIZING HAND PULL
1 page 22
2 page 22

> LIMBERING ELBOW CIRCLES
3 page 23
4 page 23

> ARTICULATING RIB BREATH
5 page 24
6 page 24

> OPENING SEATED CAT
11 page 27
12 page 27

> ELONGATING SHOULDER WEDGE
15 page 29
16 page 29

> OPENING ARM FANS
19 page 31
20 page 31

> POWERING MODIFIED COBRA
21 page 32
22 page 32

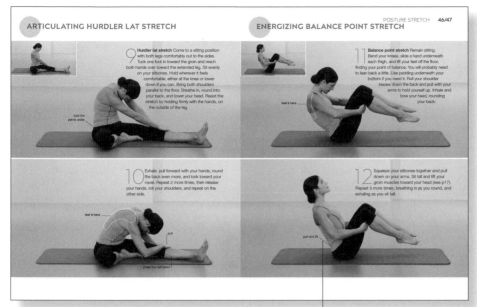

"Feel-it-here" outlines in some of the illustrations to the steps reveal the particular areas of your body that the stretch is working on—and where you are most likely to feel the benefits.

annotations provide extra cues, tips, and insights

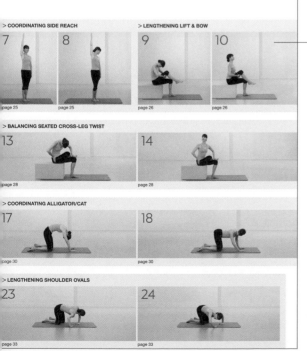

the summary shows all the exercises in the program

At-a-glance summaries demonstrate the flow of each program, providing a quick reference so that you can perform a neat, succinct, 15-minute sequence.

DEFINING THE STRETCH

Welcome to the world of stretching. Not only will you come across many stretches, you will also find many types of stretches. Forget all those preconceived notions about the value of holding a stretch for an indefinite amount of time. Let these stretches move you.

There's more than one way to stretch. That's because there's more to it than simply stretching muscles. Arteries, veins, and nerves that supply the muscles are involved, too. What is also important is the stretch of the fascia—the connective tissue that permeates the whole body and wraps around the muscles and holds them close to the skeleton.

Think of it as a biomechanical "architecture." The bones are the scaffolding and the fascia is the bricks and mortar that support the volume of the structure. The fascia adapts to its environment. If you were put into a small closet and forced to sit in a crouched position for days on end, over time your body would attempt to shrink to fit into the extreme environment. The fascia does the same.

TYPES OF STRETCHING

- **Re-coordination stretches** increase range by changing repetitive motor patterns caused by right or left dominance.

- **Reciprocal stretches** use the natural shortening and lengthening effect on either side of a joint to create more stretch.

- **Fascial stretches** focus on the fascia and help to balance muscle connections; they are particularly effective for opening and stretching the torso.

COMPENSATING FOR BAD HABITS

Our bodies are remarkably forgiving because we still function, even with poor posture—rounded shoulders and a forward head, or a protruding belly or collapsing ankles. The body compensates for weaknesses or faulty habits, but the compensations become "solidified," altering the patterns of our fascia and muscles. For this reason, we need different types of stretching to reverse any tightening to which our body has become accustomed.

STRETCHING STRATEGIES

We also need different stretches to address the properties of the various parts of our body. Moving stretches where, for instance, the head is rotating, the knee is bending, or the arm is circling, tend to be re-coordination stretches. They help to break up the body patterns we develop from being right- or left-handed, as well the patterns that come from other reoccurring motions. Merely changing the direction of those familiar patterns can significantly increase our range of motion.

Another stretching strategy has to do with stretching muscles on the opposite side of joints. This is called reciprocal stretching. For instance, when you bend your elbow, the muscles on the front side of the joint—the biceps—shorten, and those on the other side—the triceps—have to lengthen to allow the motion. Using reciprocal stretching techniques automatically relaxes the lengthening side, allowing those muscles to stretch.

STRETCHING THE FASCIA

Other types of stretches work on stretching the fascia in several ways. Stretching the spine using a breathing and rippling action helps stretch the torso from horizontal segment to horizontal segment. Another fascial stretch works on stretching the muscle connection chain that runs from the waist, down the back of the leg, and into the foot (see pp12–13). This program also includes some stretches specifically designed to glide the arm and leg nerves in their sheaths, which allows greater ease of motion. The details make the difference; read the instructions carefully to find the precision that will give you your best stretch.

The devil's in the detail. Find the precision you need for each stretch by studying the demonstrations and imagining the cues.

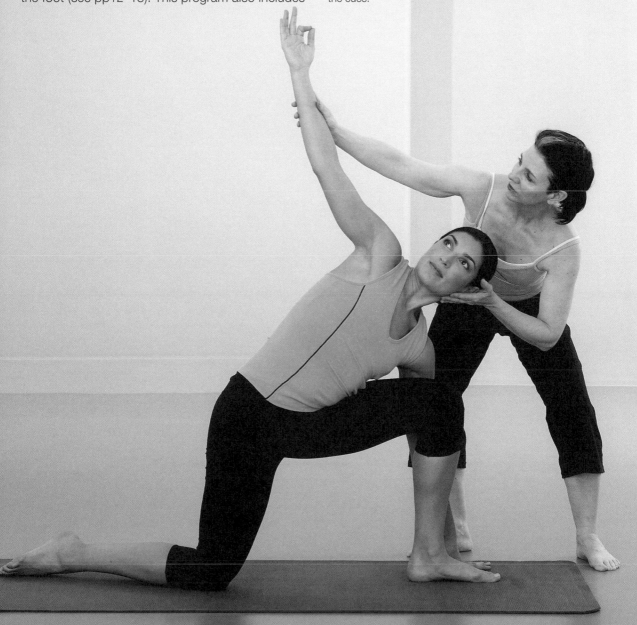

MUSCLE CONNECTIONS

Proper positioning of the arms, legs, and head helps us to physically find the link between muscle and connective tissue. Using focus and intent when we line up these extremities with the torso gives us a powerful tool for changing body posture and developing litheness.

The science of biomechanics identifies various structural body connections and physical forces that are involved in body function. In order to devise appropriate exercises, it is necessary to use our knowledge of the nature of our body parts (how plastic, or changeable, the various components are) to create the effect we need. Three important structural connections in the body that we have to consider are the "X" model, the inner unit, and the lateral system.

THE "X" MODEL
The "X" model shows the connection between what is going on externally and the inner unit (see below). It shows how the limbs are connected with each other and how these connections pass right through the inner unit. Think deep; think three-dimensional. The right arm, for example, is connected to the left leg and vice versa. The positioning of the head, which can weigh up to 15 pounds (6.8kg), is also important. Tipping it in any direction activates an intricate system of overlapping muscles that bind the head into the trunk yet allow a marvelous telescoping range to the neck.

THE INNER UNIT
Various groups of muscles form the inner unit. These are the muscles at the bottom of the torso (the pelvic floor), the deep abdominal muscles, the transverse abdominals at the sides of the abdomen, the deep low-back muscles, the multifidi (a group of muscles on either side of the spine), and the

PULLING IT ALL TOGETHER

- **Coordination** between opposing limbs and the trunk is demonstrated by the "X" model concept.

- **Precision** in stretching is created by achieving stabilization of the inner unit, which provides a firm foundation.

- **Elongation of the lateral system** promotes symmetry and balance.

muscles deep inside the rib cage (the diaphragm).

Working the muscles of the inner unit correctly—with good form—promotes low-back and pelvic health. The exercise instructions also help you use the inner unit as a stabilizing foundation, giving more precision when you stretch the external parts.

THE LATERAL SYSTEM
The lateral system connects the muscles and fascia (see p10) that run down the sides of the body. Think of it as a long road running from the triceps in the upper arm, past the armpit, down the side of the ribs and waist, extending down the side of the leg past the thigh and shin, and ending at the side of the foot. This lateral system is often overlooked, but opening it through stretching is key to balancing the body and improving posture.

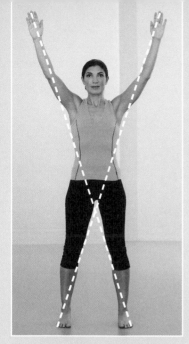

The "X" model shows the link between what goes on internally and externally. Opposite sides of the body criss-cross, attaching the limbs and head to the torso.

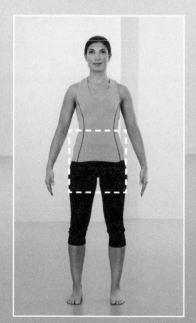

The inner unit is the foundation of our body. It houses our center of gravity. Anchoring this area provides a counterbalance to, and increased effectiveness for, each stretch.

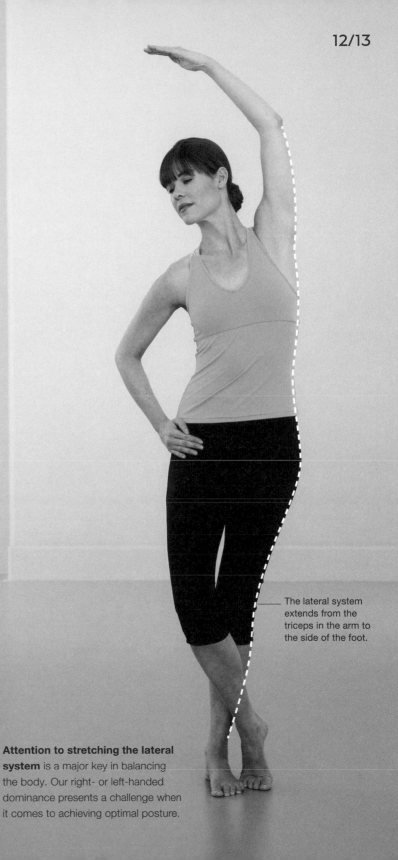

The lateral system extends from the triceps in the arm to the side of the foot.

Attention to stretching the lateral system is a major key in balancing the body. Our right- or left-handed dominance presents a challenge when it comes to achieving optimal posture.

FLEXIBILITY AND POSTURE

Genetics dictate how flexible you are and also your postural body type. Stiffness and over-flexibility both cause aches, pains, and difficulty in day-to-day activities. Explore your flexibility with these easy tests, and strive to find your best neutral posture.

Gravity has a greater impact upon our posture when we are upright in sitting or standing. If we give in to it, the "segments" of our body collapse (see below left). The result is that our muscles are out of balance and our joints are misaligned.

Stretching counterbalances this and helps you develop a good neutral posture. You start by using good form and working the muscles of the inner unit (see p12). This helps you stretch the chest and shorten the upper back muscles, open the low back and engage the abs, as well as stretch the front of the hips and thighs, and the calves.

Practicing sitting and standing tall also solidifies our intent to push vertically upward against the force of gravity. The beauty of this formula is that it applies to all body types and levels of flexibility, even people who are naturally flexible.

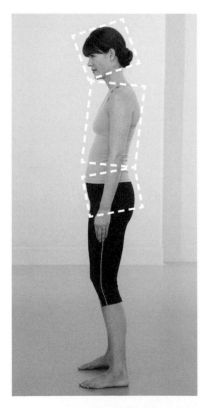 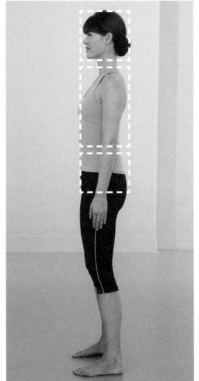

Gravity breaks us into unbalanced segments (far left). The head falls forward. The chest shortens and sinks, and the upper back rounds. The low back tightens and collapses, and the abdomen protrudes. The front of the thighs and hips tighten, while the hip extensors slacken. Body weight lists back on the heels, shortening the calves.

The goal is to balance the segments and achieve neutral posture, with a straight line running from the head through the pelvis (left). Note especially how the weight of the heavy head is now balanced directly over the pelvis, which houses our center of gravity. This alignment puts the least amount of strain on the spine as well as the other joints in the body.

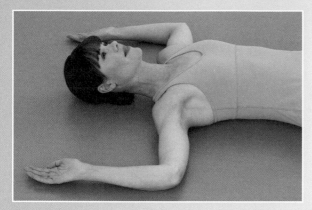

Test the mobility of your shoulders and upper back. Lie on the floor with your arms bent and your forearms parallel with the sides of you head. Your muscles are over-tight if your head and forearms do not touch the floor.

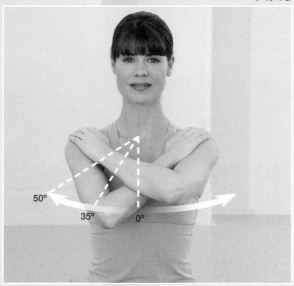

50° 35° 0°

Test the mobility of your spine, rib cage, and neck. From a seated position, cross your arms, put each hand on the opposite shoulder, and rotate your torso. Note how far you can go. Anything less than 35° indicates that your muscles are over-tight. Being right-handed or left-handed affects how far you can rotate.

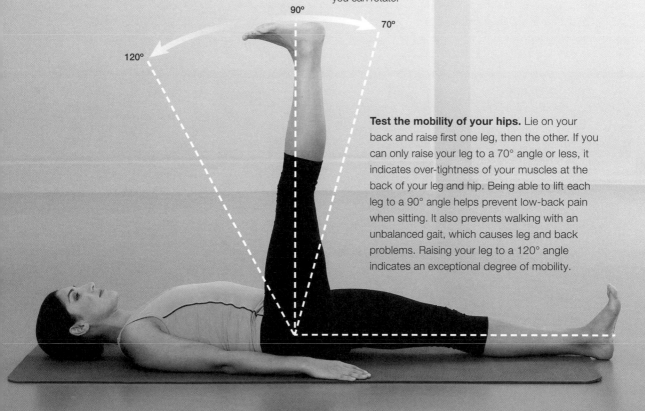

120° 90° 70°

Test the mobility of your hips. Lie on your back and raise first one leg, then the other. If you can only raise your leg to a 70° angle or less, it indicates over-tightness of your muscles at the back of your leg and hip. Being able to lift each leg to a 90° angle helps prevent low-back pain when sitting. It also prevents walking with an unbalanced gait, which causes leg and back problems. Raising your leg to a 120° angle indicates an exceptional degree of mobility.

IMAGERY AS A TOOL

Use imagery as a tool to help create precision and a sense of the inner layers of your body in your stretches. Connecting everyday concepts to the exercises gives your stretches an effective edge. Strive to internalize the cues. They hold the key to true physical transformation.

Actors, musicians, and dancers use imagery to help them "act out" their message. Children play imaginary roles in imaginary settings to prepare for adult life. As adults, we can employ imagery to help us make our exercise more effective.

The exercise programs in this book contain some imagery cues that ask you to use your imagination. Focus on them to help coordinate your muscles and access the deeper connections of your body. For example, "Lift the imaginary swimming-pool water" asks you to press upward in the abdomen when you're lying on your front. Mention of "smile lines" is a cue for you to hold your hips in true extension when lying down, and give you the range of motion you need to achieve a neutral pelvis. When you get it right, two arcs separate the buttocks from the upper thighs or hamstrings (see below).

By training these deeper muscles to engage as you perform your stretching exercises, you also train them to engage when you carry out your everyday activities. Although some images apply to certain body positions, such as finding the smile lines while lying on your front, you can also relate to them in other positions. In other words, you can find your smile lines when you're standing, too. They can help you find your neutral posture (see p14).

The imagery I use is truly the key to taking your exercise life into your daily life. Study the pictures in the exercises on these two pages, and start a lifelong habit of using your body more completely.

Imagining water pushing up against the abdomen deepens abdominal connections. Visualizing "smile lines" stabilizes the pelvis and brings precision into hip stretches.

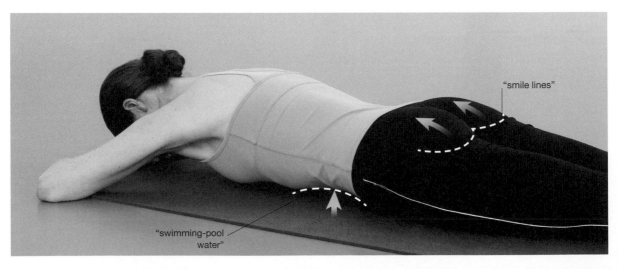

"smile lines"

"swimming-pool water"

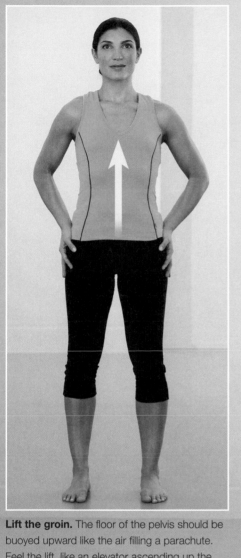

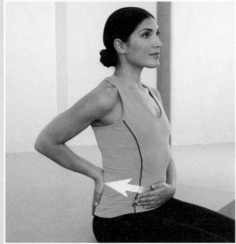

Preserve your natural low-back curve by sitting forward on your sitbones. Simultaneously pull the navel to the spine to sandwich the waist with a corset of muscles.

Coordinate the stretch between your head and legs. Reach your head out of the collarbones, like a turtle reaching its head out of a shell. At the same time, balance and reach out through the top foot.

Lift the groin. The floor of the pelvis should be buoyed upward like the air filling a parachute. Feel the lift, like an elevator ascending up the spine toward the head.

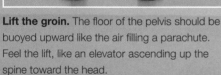

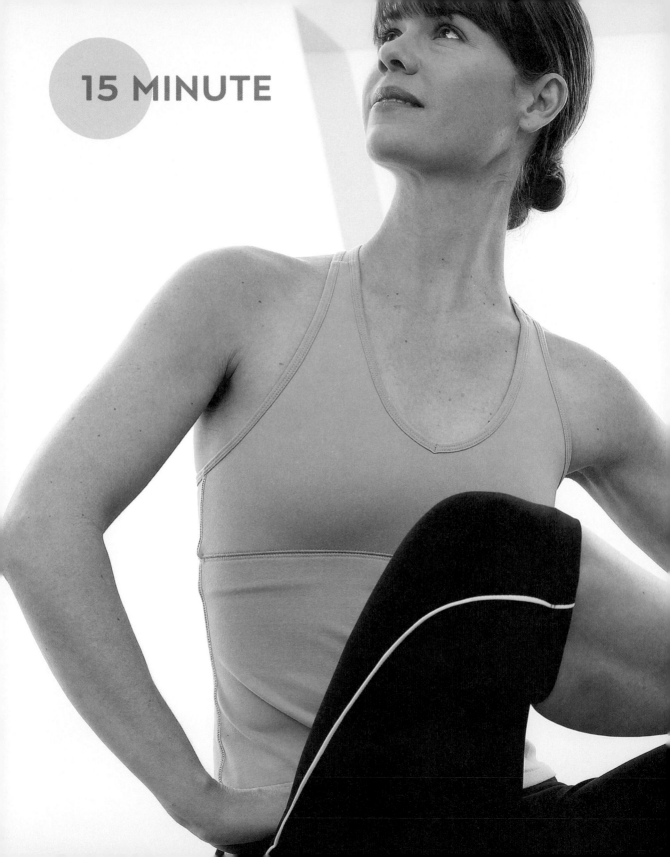

15 MINUTE

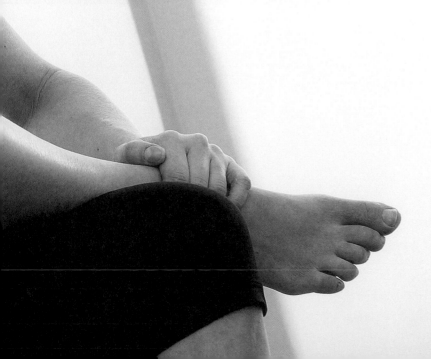

WAKE UP
THE STRETCH

START TO MASTER YOUR STRETCH
THINK THREE-DIMENSIONALLY
FOCUS ON BODY SENSATIONS
BREATHE SMOOTHLY AND DEEPLY

WAKE UP THE STRETCH

Your stretch journey starts with a sequence that creates suppleness and wakes up your stretch. No matter what your level, as you stretch your whole body, you'll find the fluid motion of this sequence as slinky as a long cat yawn. Try to imagine that you're "connecting the dots" as you weave your way through each and every movement.

Stretching is a skill that everyone can master. This sequence emphasizes the various techniques you'll need and the sensory elements of stretch that together will help make your stretch possible. Being able to identify muscle tone is a crucial first step. Next, learning to stabilize one part of the body while another moves away from the stabilizing part is key to the effectiveness of a lengthening stretch. Breathing into tight body areas such as the back of the rib cage demands discipline and focus. Loosening and circling motions help oil the joints and loosen restrictive connective tissue, prompting muscles to expand and contract. Re-coordination exercises (see p10) make new ranges of motion possible for everyone.

THE EXERCISES

Feel as much of your body as you can in the Hand Pull. Memorize this muscular feeling and strive to carry that feeling into the rest of the sequence. Make the Elbow Circles as sensory and luscious as if you were moving through a pool of honey. Direct the flow of your breath very specifically into any tight parts of the diaphragm. This exercise may feel difficult at first, but it can give you a very satisfying sense of relaxation.

The seated exercises may seem easy, but use the surface and structure of the chair to explore your orientation in space. Notice the relationship among your hip, rib, head, arm, and leg placements. The physical boundary of the chair not only provides landmarks so you can judge how far a stretch is

TIPS FOR WAKE UP THE STRETCH

- **Internalize your stretches** by giving as much detailed focus to your body sensations as possible.

- **Try to imagine** the infrastructure—the skeletal part that is moving—such as your arms moving against your upper torso.

- **Work to identify** which parts are anchoring and which parts are moving.

- **Strive to feel the entire path of the motion,** not just the end points.

- **Breathe in long, flowing, time-released breaths,** as suggested by the guide music; be sure not to hold your breath.

moving, it can also give you a sense of your deep muscles, which can help if you feel your movement is restricted. Sitting on a firm surface is also a sneaky way to feel some input up into your sitbones. This pressure gives a neurological stimulus to your "righting" reflex, which helps you lengthen up against gravity. The Seated Cross-leg Twist and Shoulder Wedge also show you how to press one body part against another to increase the stretch, as well as adding a strengthening element to your stretches.

On the other end of the scale are the Shoulder Ovals. They demonstrate an instance where learning to respect a joint's boundary is of great importance, since neck, arms, and shoulders tend to be more sensitive to injury thanks to their potential for extreme movement. The Shoulder Ovals also provide a superb nerve stretch and glide—a nerve glide being a movement that creates frictionless motion of the nerve. This, ultimately, will increase the range of movement of the whole of your upper body.

Simple stretching positions while sitting can bring about big changes when you perform them with coordination, precision, and intent.

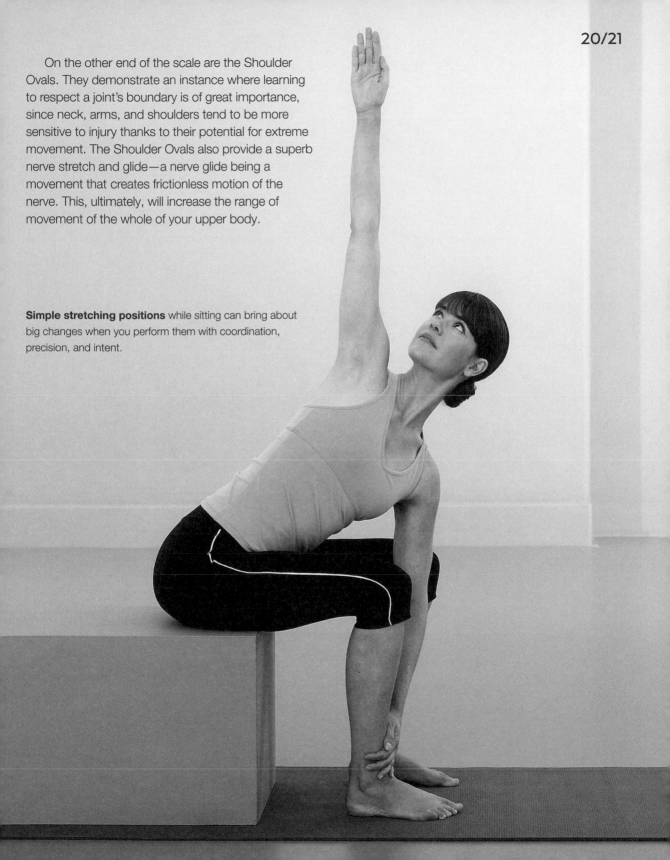

ENERGIZING HAND PULL

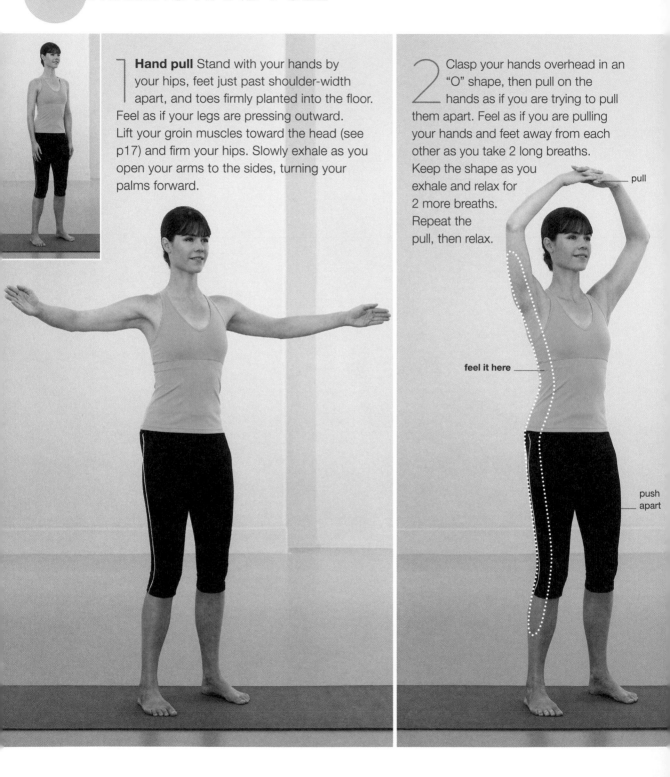

1 Hand pull Stand with your hands by your hips, feet just past shoulder-width apart, and toes firmly planted into the floor. Feel as if your legs are pressing outward. Lift your groin muscles toward the head (see p17) and firm your hips. Slowly exhale as you open your arms to the sides, turning your palms forward.

2 Clasp your hands overhead in an "O" shape, then pull on the hands as if you are trying to pull them apart. Feel as if you are pulling your hands and feet away from each other as you take 2 long breaths. Keep the shape as you exhale and relax for 2 more breaths. Repeat the pull, then relax.

pull

feel it here

push apart

LIMBERING ELBOW CIRCLES

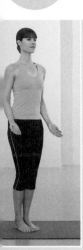

3 **Elbow circles** Bring your feet and inner thighs completely together and place your hands at your hips, with your palms facing forward. Inhale, and fold your elbows to take your fingertips to your shoulders, pointing the elbows forward.

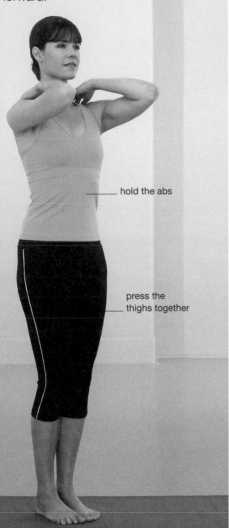

hold the abs

press the thighs together

4 Exhale, lift the elbows, and smoothly circle the hands up and diagonally behind you. Repeat 3 more times.

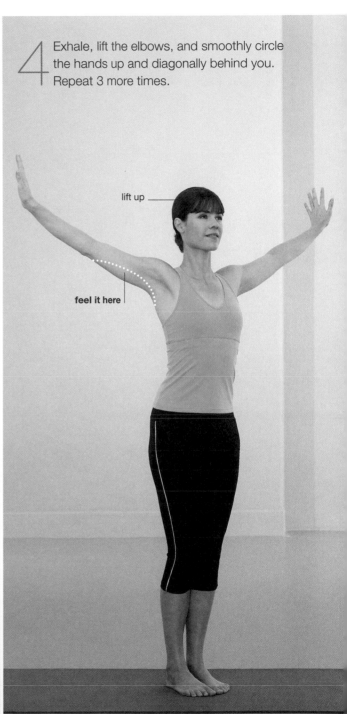

lift up

feel it here

ARTICULATING RIB BREATH

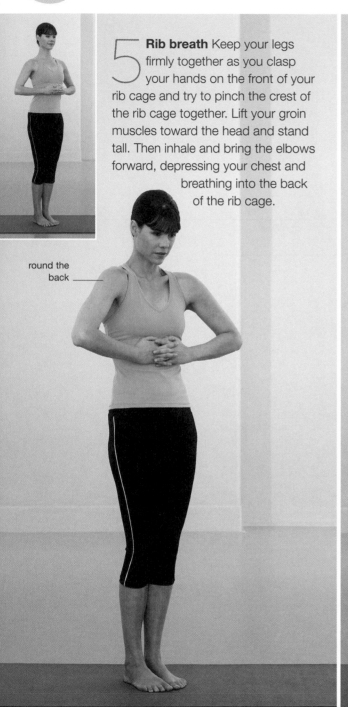

5 **Rib breath** Keep your legs firmly together as you clasp your hands on the front of your rib cage and try to pinch the crest of the rib cage together. Lift your groin muscles toward the head and stand tall. Then inhale and bring the elbows forward, depressing your chest and breathing into the back of the rib cage.

round the back

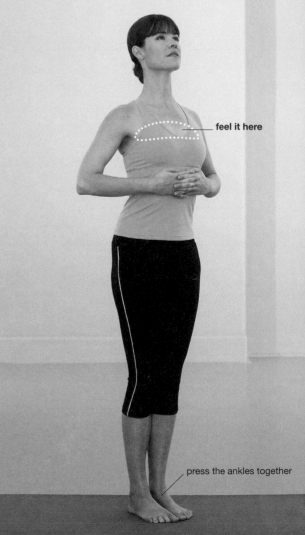

6 Reverse the movement. Exhale, open the chest, lengthen up through your head, and look diagonally upward. Allow your elbows to come backward. Repeat 2 more times, inhaling as you bring the elbows forward, and exhaling as you open the chest. Release your hands and shake them gently to release any tension in them.

feel it here

press the ankles together

COORDINATING SIDE REACH

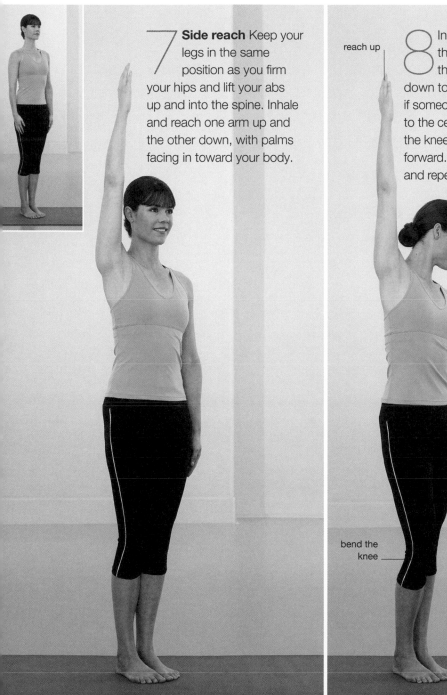

7 **Side reach** Keep your legs in the same position as you firm your hips and lift your abs up and into the spine. Inhale and reach one arm up and the other down, with palms facing in toward your body.

reach up

8 Intensify the stretch by bending the knee slightly on the side of the raised hand and by looking down toward the lower hand. Feel as if someone is pulling your middle finger to the ceiling. Then exhale, straighten the knee, and slowly turn your face forward. Repeat, then change sides and repeat 2 times on the other side. Let your arm come down and relax.

look down

bend the knee

LENGTHENING LIFT & BOW

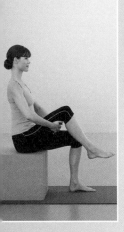

9 **Lift & bow** Sit on the edge of a chair with your feet hip-width apart. Feel your sitbones pressing equally on the seat. Sit tall, lift your groin muscles toward your head, then hold onto one thigh and lift the knee toward the ceiling. Inhale, then lift up into your waist and bow your head toward your knee.

10 Exhale and reverse, lifting your chest and face diagonally up toward the ceiling. Repeat 2 more times, inhaling as you bow, and exhaling as you lift. Lower the foot to the floor and repeat on the other side.

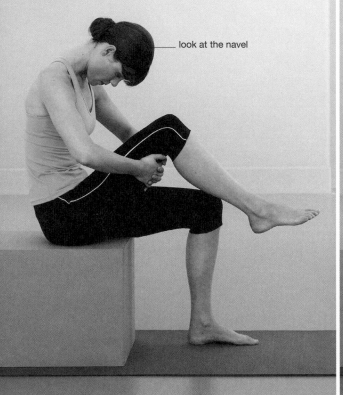

look at the navel

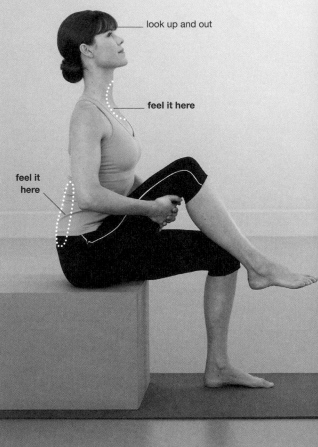

look up and out

feel it here

feel it here

OPENING SEATED CAT

11 **Seated cat** Remain sitting toward the edge of your seat. Extend one foot out on the floor in front of you, keeping the knee a little bent, and pressing the sole and big toe of the foot firmly on the floor. Place your hands on the same thigh. Inhale as you round your back.

12 Exhale and reverse the curve. Start from the lower back, and move through the middle and upper back with a ripple effect to lift the chest and face diagonally toward the ceiling. Inhale, round and repeat, then repeat the whole stretch on the other side. Roll your shoulders and release.

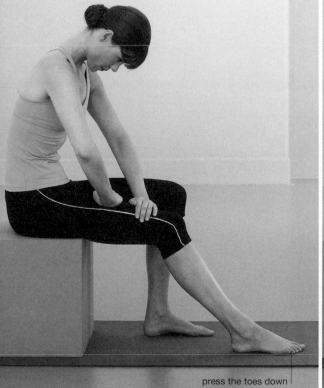

press the toes down

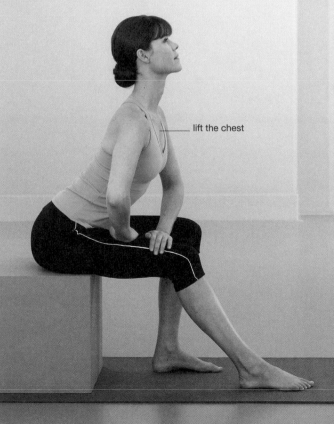

lift the chest

BALANCING SEATED CROSS-LEG TWIST

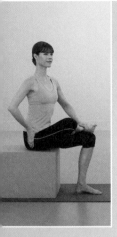

13 **Seated cross-leg twist** Remain seated, cross one foot on top of the opposite thigh, and hold onto your ankle with the other hand. Place the same hand as your crossed leg on your hip. Inhale, lift your groin muscles toward the head, lengthen your spine, and bow your head toward your knee.

14 Exhale, lift your chest, and turn your torso toward your crossed leg. Look past your shoulder. Repeat 2 more times, inhaling as you bow and exhaling as you lift, then repeat 3 times on the other side. Slowly release the leg, come out of the position, and gently move your back to release any tension.

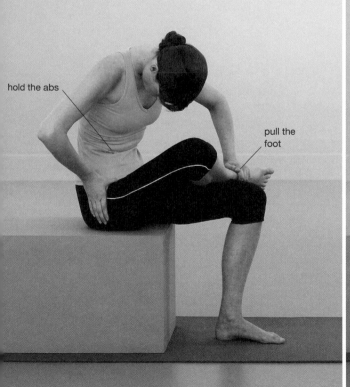

hold the abs

pull the foot

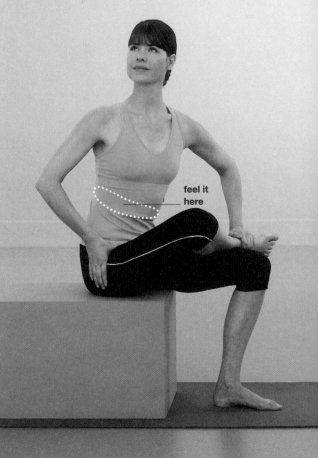

feel it here

ELONGATING SHOULDER WEDGE

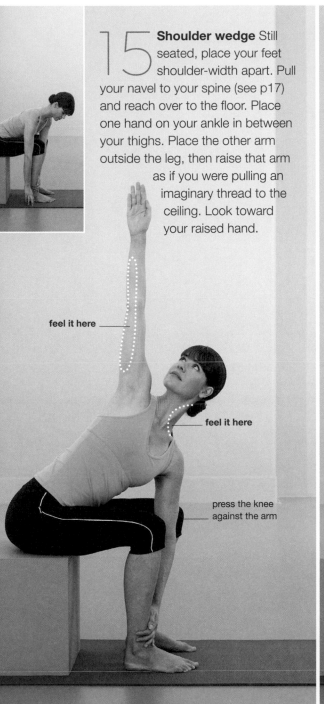

15 **Shoulder wedge** Still seated, place your feet shoulder-width apart. Pull your navel to your spine (see p17) and reach over to the floor. Place one hand on your ankle in between your thighs. Place the other arm outside the leg, then raise that arm as if you were pulling an imaginary thread to the ceiling. Look toward your raised hand.

feel it here

feel it here

press the knee against the arm

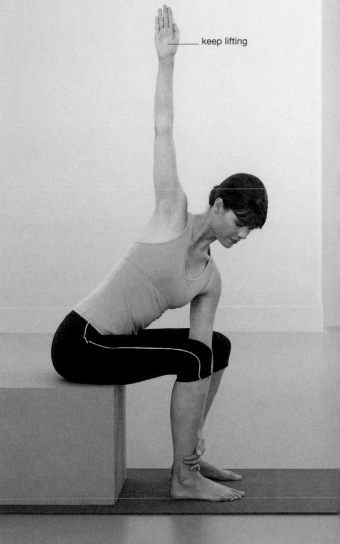

16 Exhale, keep your arm lifted, and consciously rotate your neck as you look down. Repeat 2 more times, inhaling as you look up, and exhaling as you look down. Bring the arm down and repeat 3 times on the other side. Roll to sit up. Take a deep breath, and relax.

keep lifting

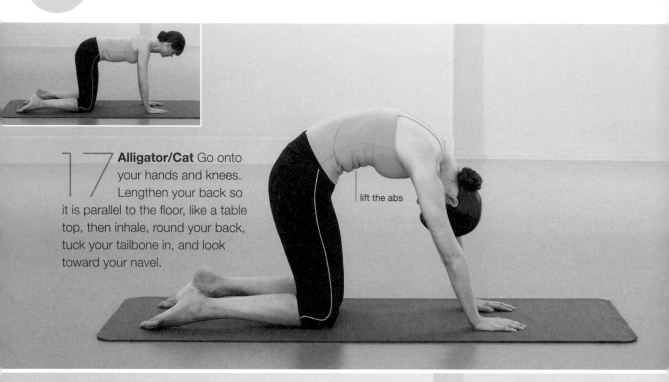

17 **Alligator/Cat** Go onto your hands and knees. Lengthen your back so it is parallel to the floor, like a table top, then inhale, round your back, tuck your tailbone in, and look toward your navel.

lift the abs

18 Exhale, lengthen your back, then sway your hips and head toward each other. Repeat on the other side, always inhaling as you round your back and exhaling as you take your hips and head toward each other. Repeat 1 more time on each side.

sway the hips toward the face

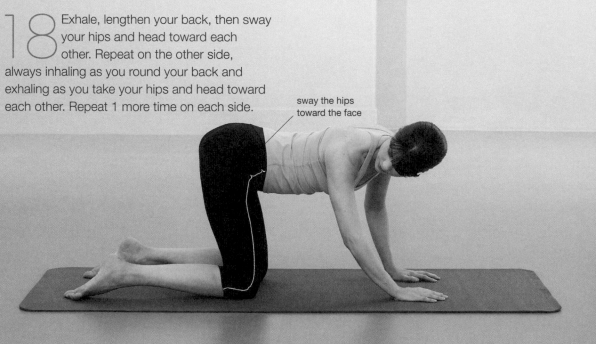

OPENING ARM FANS

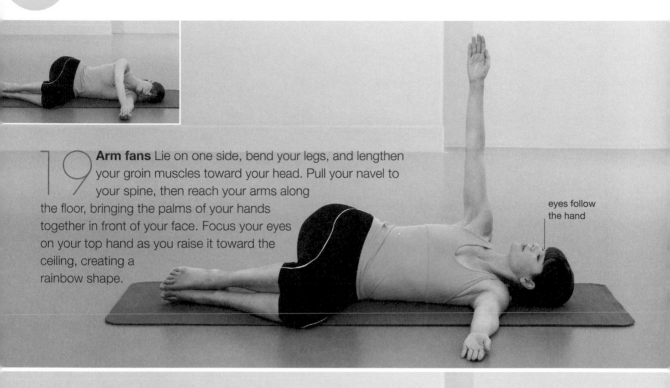

19 **Arm fans** Lie on one side, bend your legs, and lengthen your groin muscles toward your head. Pull your navel to your spine, then reach your arms along the floor, bringing the palms of your hands together in front of your face. Focus your eyes on your top hand as you raise it toward the ceiling, creating a rainbow shape.

eyes follow the hand

20 Continue moving the arm and reach behind you to the floor, allowing your shoulders and torso to rotate with the arm. Try not to move your knees. Exhale, then reach up with the hand as you reverse, "painting the ceiling" with your fingertips until your hands are together again. Repeat 2 more times, inhaling as you open the arm, exhaling as you bring the palms together again. Roll over to the other side and repeat.

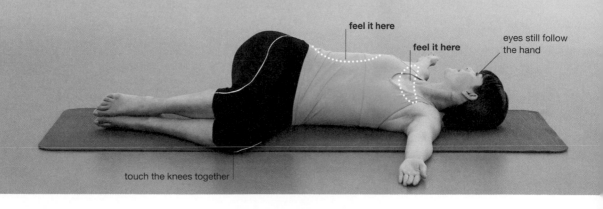

feel it here

feel it here

eyes still follow the hand

touch the knees together

POWERING MODIFIED COBRA

21 **Modified cobra** Go onto your stomach, firm and tighten your hips, and feel the smile lines (see p16) between your glutes and your hamstrings. Lift the groin muscles toward the head. Feel the imaginary swimming-pool water lifting your abdomen off the floor (see p16). Reach your hands out onto the floor in front of you.

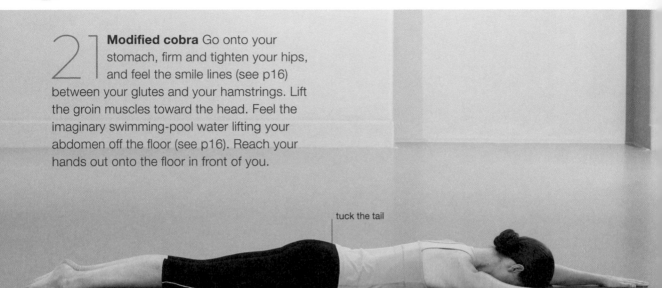

tuck the tail

lift the abs

22 Inhale as you drag your hands along the floor toward your shoulders, keeping the abdomen tight and lifting your front body so your ribs come off the floor. Exhale, slide the arms out in front of you, and take your face back to the floor. Repeat, then relax and breathe normally.

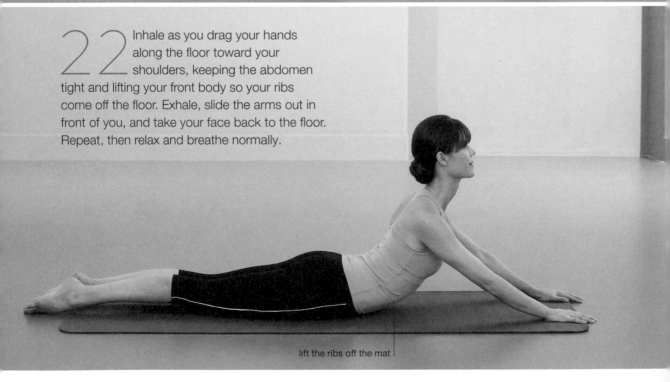

lift the ribs off the mat

LENGTHENING SHOULDER OVALS

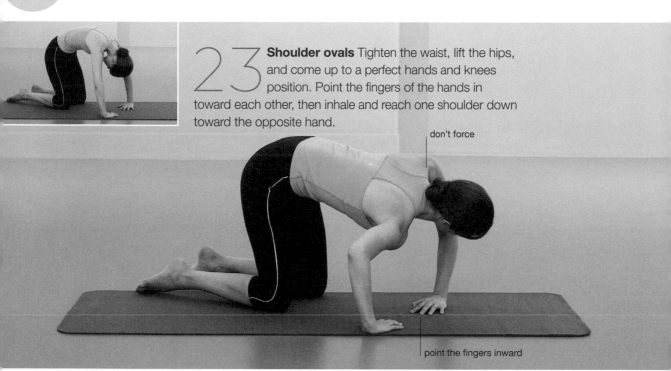

23 **Shoulder ovals** Tighten the waist, lift the hips, and come up to a perfect hands and knees position. Point the fingers of the hands in toward each other, then inhale and reach one shoulder down toward the opposite hand.

don't force

point the fingers inward

24 Sweep the chest across the floor, past center toward the other hand, then exhale and continue circling in the same direction as you round your back. Your shoulders should be describing an oval in space. Keep going in the same direction for 2 more ovals, then change direction and reverse for 2 more ovals.

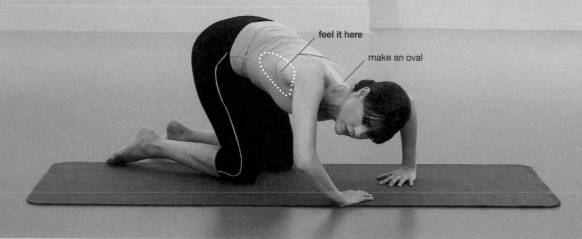

feel it here

make an oval

WAKE UP THE STRETCH AT A GLANCE

> ENERGIZING HAND PULL

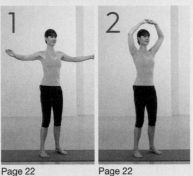

1

Page 22

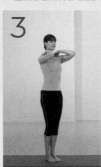

2

Page 22

> LIMBERING ELBOW CIRCLES

3

Page 23

4

Page 23

> ARTICULATING RIB BREATH

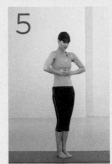

5

Page 24

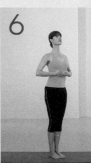

6

Page 24

> OPENING SEATED CAT

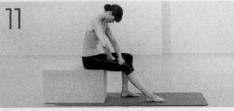

11

Page 27

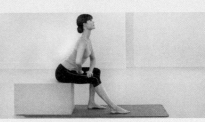

12

Page 27

> ELONGATING SHOULDER WEDGE

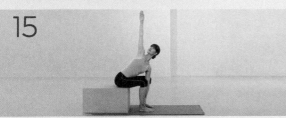

15

Page 29

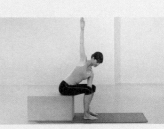

16

Page 29

> OPENING ARM FANS

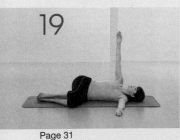

19

Page 31

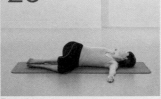

20

Page 31

> POWERING MODIFIED COBRA

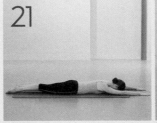

21

Page 32

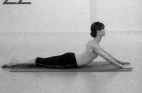

22

Page 32

> **COORDINATING SIDE REACH**

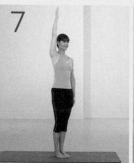 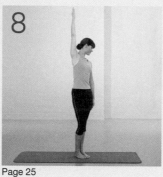

Page 25   Page 25

> **LENGTHENING LIFT & BOW**

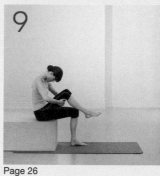 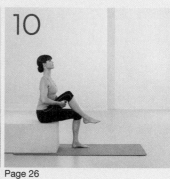

Page 26   Page 26

> **BALANCING SEATED CROSS-LEG TWIST**

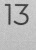 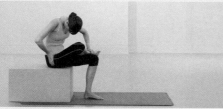

Page 28   Page 28

> **COORDINATING ALLIGATOR/CAT**

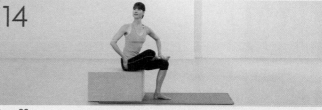 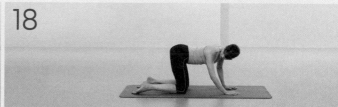

Page 30   Page 30

> **LENGTHENING SHOULDER OVALS**

 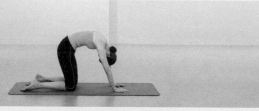 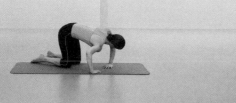 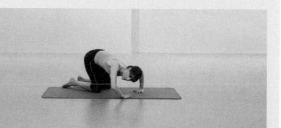

Page 33   Page 33

WAKE UP THE STRETCH FAQS

The Wake Up the Stretch program is excellent for beginners as well as for someone looking for a lighter, more gentle stretch. During this first program, learn to create focus by coordinating inner and outer muscles through the use of the cues and imagery.

HOW IS THE HAND PULL A STRETCH?

This overhead pull is a sneaky way to stretch the sides of the torso, especially around the armpits, as well as stretching the sides of the hips and legs. Some people will not be able even to reach their hands together in an overhead position, so this exercise makes a great starting point. It's possible that one half of your pelvis is tighter than the other. As you push the legs away from each other, you are beginning to equalize each side, balancing right with left.

IN THE RIB BREATH EXERCISE, IT SEEMS AS IF NOTHING IS MOVING. WHAT CAN I DO?

You have to have faith that something is happening. The deep connective tissue and the big domelike breathing muscle, the diaphragm, tend to be tight in the back of the rib cage on most people. It's a lot easier to see movement in the front part. Try coughing or sniffing repetitively; feel the action of the diaphragm and ribs in the front. It's anatomically not possible to have a great deal of motion in the back, but in this exercise we begin by cinching the front of the dome, which forces the back to stretch.

HOW DO I KNOW I'M DOING THE SIDE REACH CORRECTLY?

First be sure you are following the instructions correctly. You have to pull upward very strongly with the armpit, arm, and hand while you bend your knee. It's not going to be a comfortable feeling once you add the turn of the head. The purpose of this exercise is to start opening the rib cage, neck, and shoulders. This is a very dense area and it's hard to tease apart the separate parts.

WHEN I'M SITTING, I CAN BARELY LIFT MY KNEE TOWARD MY HEAD IN LIFT & BOW, BUT THE MODEL'S KNEE IS ALMOST TOUCHING. AM I STILL STRETCHING?

Absolutely. The important part of this stretch is the lengthening and softening of the spine. I jokingly call this "marinating" the spine. Moving the head up and down also helps to move the spinal cord, which is healthy for the nervous system. Think of it as flossing your nerves. They need to stretch and glide, too.

THE MODEL IN THE MODIFIED COBRA IS GETTING WAY MORE OFF OF THE FLOOR THAN I AM. DOES IT MATTER?

Again, less can be more in this instance, too. Intent goes a long way when we are meeting the boundaries of our limitations. The whole idea is to find out how far you can go in a certain direction. Honor that limitation; don't force it. But meet the boundary, watch the model, and think of the direction of the motion, not so much the endpoint.

THE SHOULDER OVALS ARE CONFUSING. HOW DO I START?

This is an extremely effective exercise for the nerves of the arms and neck. Many people don't realize how much restriction they have in their shoulders until they develop a problem. So persist. Start slow. Follow the exact instructions. Sometimes it's helpful to brace your hands on a table and start there first to get the idea of the flow of the movement. Precision is best, but sometimes you just have to gyrate a bit first.

MY BACK DOESN'T MAKE A ROUND SHAPE LIKE THE MODEL'S IN THE ALLIGATOR/CAT. WHAT SHOULD I DO?

Have faith. Rome wasn't built in a day. Just by attempting the exercise and imagining the shapes you will begin, little by little, to loosen up your back. After just a few weeks, you'll notice your back will feel better and you'll be able to bend and move more easily in everyday life.

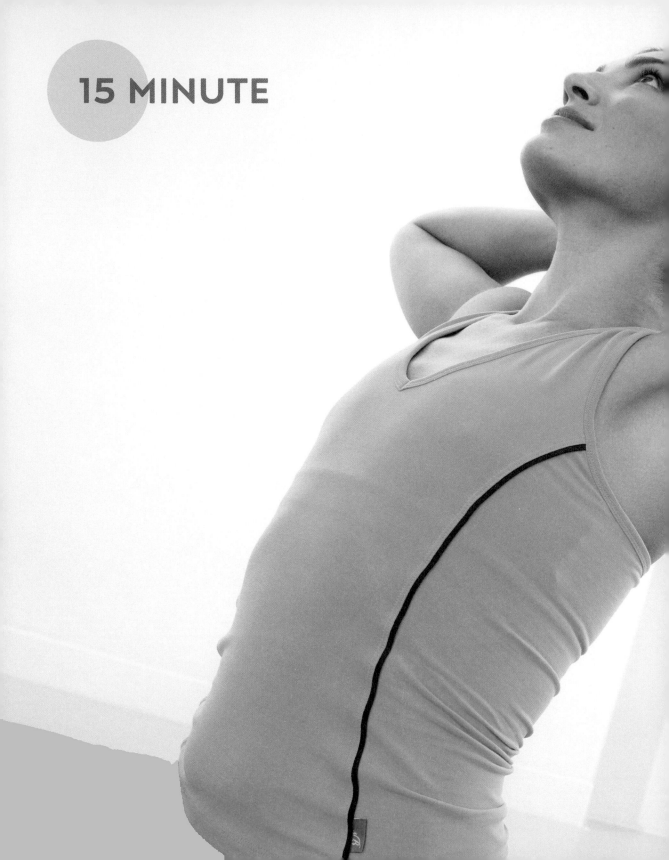

15 MINUTE

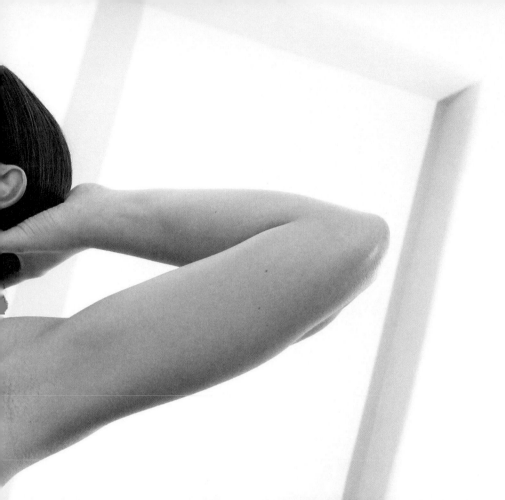

POSTURE STRETCH

FIND YOUR CENTER
ELONGATE YOUR WAIST
EXTEND UP AGAINST THE FORCE OF GRAVITY

POSTURE STRETCH

We all desire healthy posture. Although we live in an imperfect world, nearly perfect posture can be achieved by methodically balancing our bodies against gravity's pull. Where the body leads, the mind goes. Improving posture will uplift your outlook on life as well as give you confidence and endurance against everyday stresses.

Stretching for healthy posture means fighting against the pull of gravity. If we do not work against gravity's pull, then the longer we live, the more bent and deformed we become. A typical gravitational pull creates a forward-jutting chin, a tight chest, and rounded shoulders. Carrying on down the body, the abdomen becomes lax and the low back becomes tighter. A domino effect continues on into the legs, shortening the front of the thighs and creating a loose area around the glutes. The end-result is an off-center line, with tight calves causing the body weight to fall back into the heels (see p14). It's no wonder joints wear out before their time. We're all living longer, so our joints—which are a key factor in our quality of life—are important to us. The value of healthy posture cannot be stressed too much. Not only do we achieve a pleasing cosmetic effect by standing upright, we also increase our vitality, since standing well promotes optimal lung capacity, which provides more oxygen for the brain to function well.

(see p14)

TIPS FOR POSTURE STRETCH

- **Focus on the ultimate goal** of elongating your entire body in every exercise.

- **Notice how each exercise builds** toward firm, upright posture.

- **Modify when needed.** Be sensible and use extra padding under the knees if they are tender.

- **Enhance balance** by focusing your eyes on a fixed object or by holding onto furniture, if necessary.

- **In the final standing exercise,** focus first on stretching out and elongating your waist as you lengthen your ribs up and off the pelvis; locate your head weight over the center of gravity in the pelvic bowl.

THE EXERCISES

The Posture Stretch sequence follows a muscle-balancing formula as well as reinforces the neurodevelopmental sequence—in other words, the basic movement patterns that get an infant from lying down to standing and walking. The Posture Stretch sequence uses all the positions that infants must achieve on their journey to walking.

Starting with exercises lying on the back, trunk control is developed, which enables optimum control of the limbs. Pay special attention to the various parts of the front of the trunk in the Elongations. Notice how the "W's" exercise straightens and elongates you, combating the typical fetal curling position many adopt when asleep. Next, the Hurdler Lat Stretch balances both sides of the back of the waist. The Balance Point Stretch literally pushes the trunk and head up against gravity. Most of us don't notice how our back is pulling us down

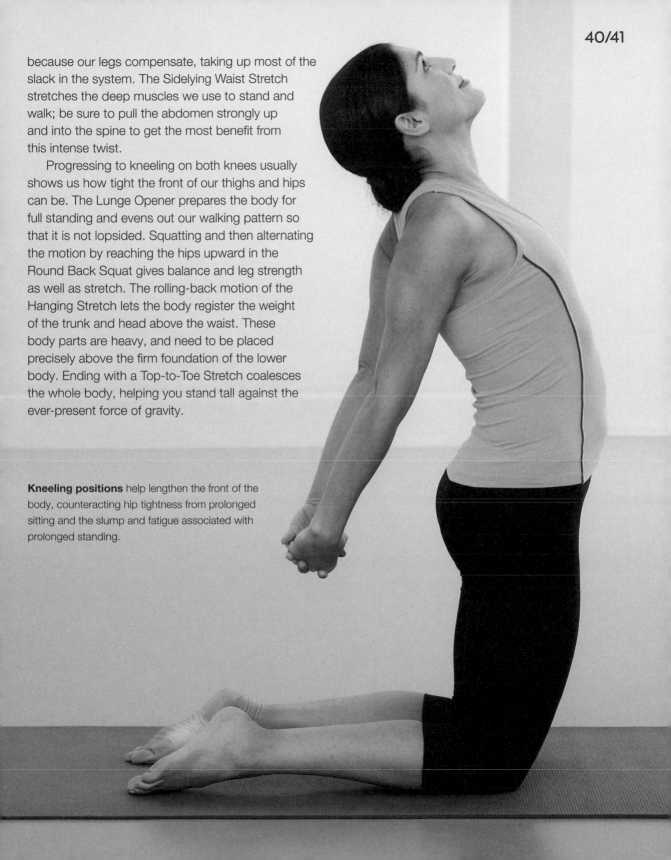

because our legs compensate, taking up most of the slack in the system. The Sidelying Waist Stretch stretches the deep muscles we use to stand and walk; be sure to pull the abdomen strongly up and into the spine to get the most benefit from this intense twist.

Progressing to kneeling on both knees usually shows us how tight the front of our thighs and hips can be. The Lunge Opener prepares the body for full standing and evens out our walking pattern so that it is not lopsided. Squatting and then alternating the motion by reaching the hips upward in the Round Back Squat gives balance and leg strength as well as stretch. The rolling-back motion of the Hanging Stretch lets the body register the weight of the trunk and head above the waist. These body parts are heavy, and need to be placed precisely above the firm foundation of the lower body. Ending with a Top-to-Toe Stretch coalesces the whole body, helping you stand tall against the ever-present force of gravity.

Kneeling positions help lengthen the front of the body, counteracting hip tightness from prolonged sitting and the slump and fatigue associated with prolonged standing.

CENTERING ELONGATIONS

1 **Elongations** Lie on your back, with your legs hip-width apart. Reach your arms beyond your head on the floor and clasp your hands. Inhale and stretch your hands and feet away from each other. Simultaneously press your low back and ribs against the floor.

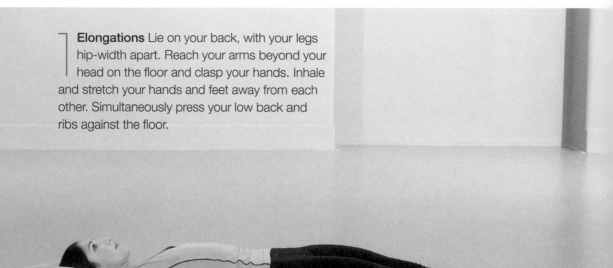

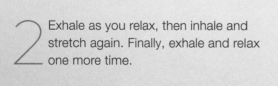

press the low back down

2 Exhale as you relax, then inhale and stretch again. Finally, exhale and relax one more time.

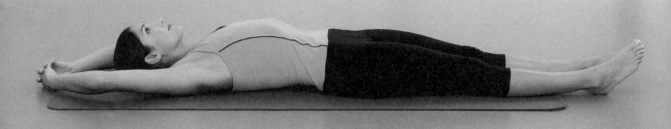

STABILIZING "W'S"

3 **"W's"** Stay on your back. Reach your arms out to the sides and bend your elbows to 90° with the backs of your hands and forearms toward the floor. If they don't touch the floor, don't force them. Inhale, then press the back of your head, forearms, shoulders, low back, and thighs into the floor.

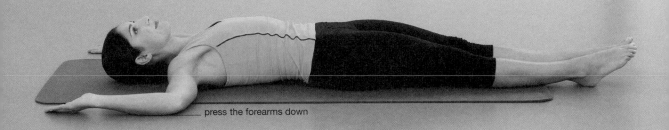

press the forearms down

4 Exhale and relax, releasing all the tension. Repeat by inhaling and pressing, and exhaling and releasing.

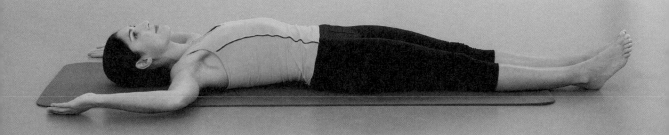

ACCENTUATING "C" STRETCH

5 **"C" stretch** Still lying on your back, reach your arms up beyond your head on the floor. Take one wrist and, keeping your shoulders against the floor, inhale and pull the wrist toward the opposite side, sliding your upper body slightly along the floor in the same direction.

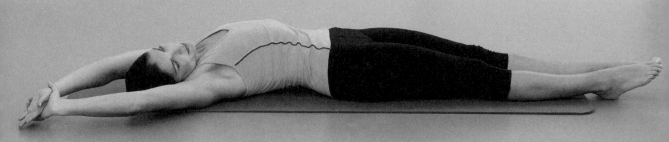

6 At the same time, cross the leg opposite to the held wrist over the other leg, and slide your legs in the same direction. This adds an extra stretch and helps to make a letter "C" with your body. Stay, inhale, and tense your abdominal muscles, then exhale and lengthen into the "C." Hold for 4 breath cycles. Lengthen and release, move back to center, and repeat on the other side. Thump the thighs to release the low back. Repeat on both sides, then thump the thighs one more time.

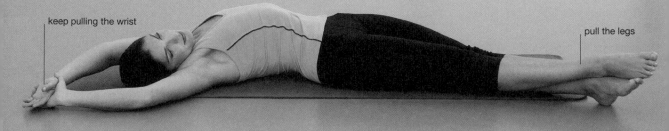

keep pulling the wrist

pull the legs

SOFTENING BABY ROCKS

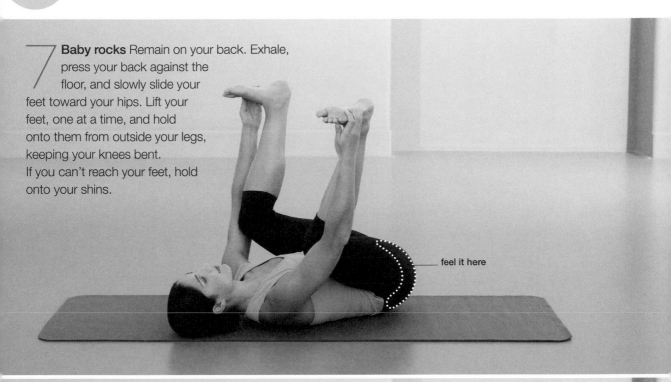

7 **Baby rocks** Remain on your back. Exhale, press your back against the floor, and slowly slide your feet toward your hips. Lift your feet, one at a time, and hold onto them from outside your legs, keeping your knees bent. If you can't reach your feet, hold onto your shins.

feel it here

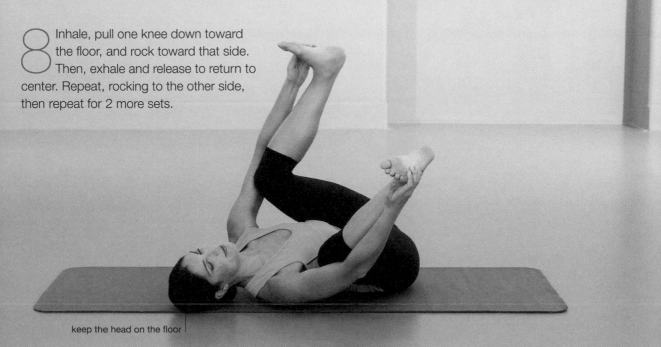

8 Inhale, pull one knee down toward the floor, and rock toward that side. Then, exhale and release to return to center. Repeat, rocking to the other side, then repeat for 2 more sets.

keep the head on the floor

ARTICULATING HURDLER LAT STRETCH

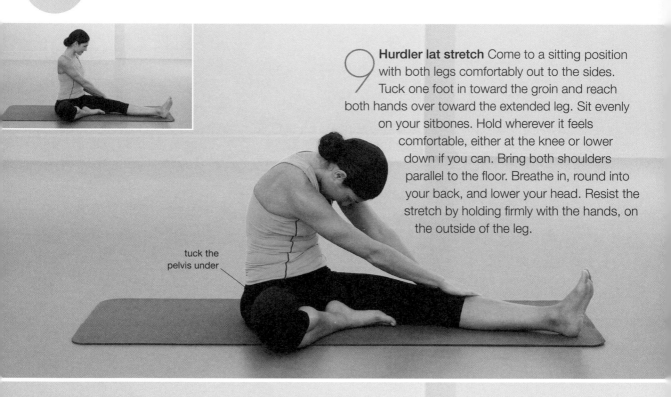

9 **Hurdler lat stretch** Come to a sitting position with both legs comfortably out to the sides. Tuck one foot in toward the groin and reach both hands over toward the extended leg. Sit evenly on your sitbones. Hold wherever it feels comfortable, either at the knee or lower down if you can. Bring both shoulders parallel to the floor. Breathe in, round into your back, and lower your head. Resist the stretch by holding firmly with the hands, on the outside of the leg.

tuck the pelvis under

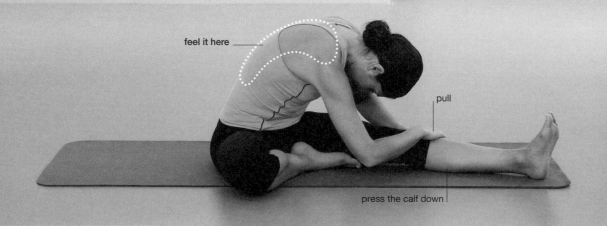

10 Exhale, pull forward with your hands, round the back even more, and look toward your navel. Repeat 2 more times, then release your hands, roll your shoulders, and repeat on the other side.

feel it here

pull

press the calf down

ENERGIZING BALANCE POINT STRETCH

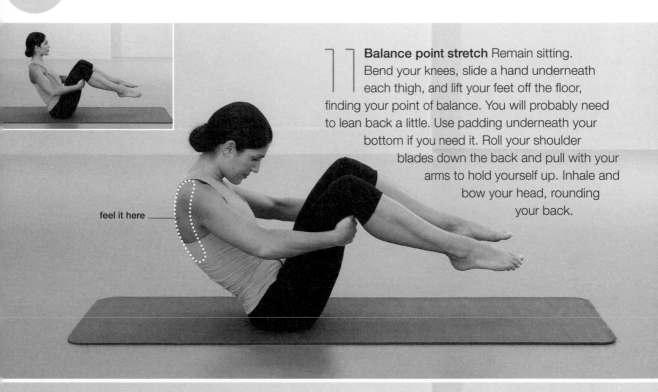

feel it here

11 **Balance point stretch** Remain sitting. Bend your knees, slide a hand underneath each thigh, and lift your feet off the floor, finding your point of balance. You will probably need to lean back a little. Use padding underneath your bottom if you need it. Roll your shoulder blades down the back and pull with your arms to hold yourself up. Inhale and bow your head, rounding your back.

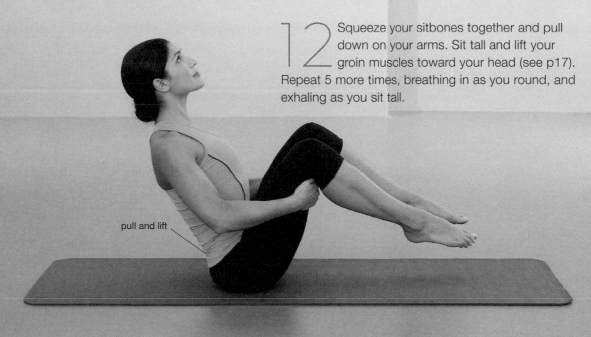

12 Squeeze your sitbones together and pull down on your arms. Sit tall and lift your groin muscles toward your head (see p17). Repeat 5 more times, breathing in as you round, and exhaling as you sit tall.

pull and lift

ELONGATING SIDELYING WAIST STRETCH

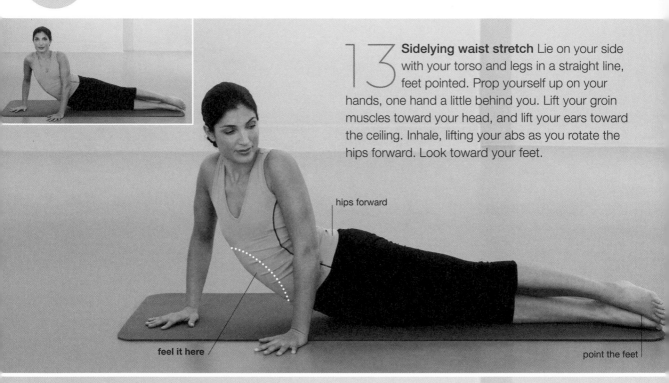

13 **Sidelying waist stretch** Lie on your side with your torso and legs in a straight line, feet pointed. Prop yourself up on your hands, one hand a little behind you. Lift your groin muscles toward your head, and lift your ears toward the ceiling. Inhale, lifting your abs as you rotate the hips forward. Look toward your feet.

hips forward

feel it here

point the feet

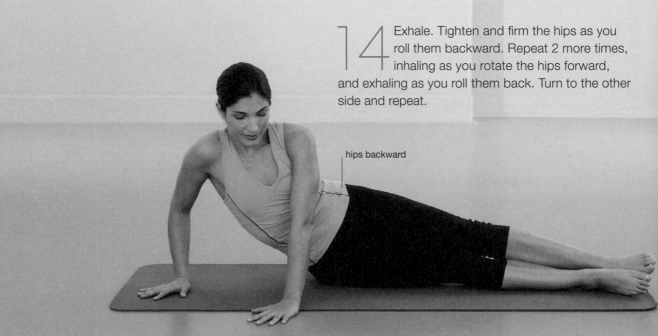

14 Exhale. Tighten and firm the hips as you roll them backward. Repeat 2 more times, inhaling as you rotate the hips forward, and exhaling as you roll them back. Turn to the other side and repeat.

hips backward

OPENING FRONT BODY OPENER

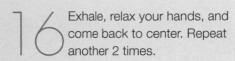

15 **Front body opener** Kneel up, with your knees under your pelvis. Use padding underneath your knees if you need it. Tuck your pelvis under and press the hips forward. Find your smile lines (see p16). Reach your arms behind you and clasp your hands behind your back, without over-arching the back. Inhale, press your hips together, and squeeze your glutes. Lift your chest and stretch your hands behind you.

16 Exhale, relax your hands, and come back to center. Repeat another 2 times.

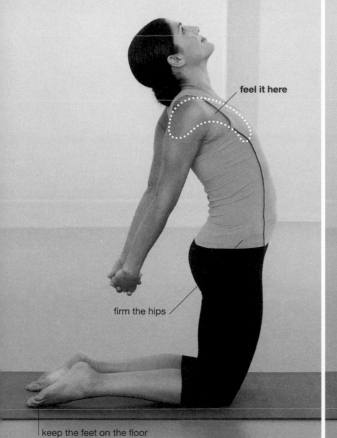

feel it here

firm the hips

keep the feet on the floor

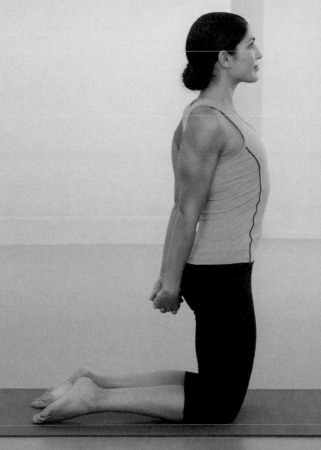

COORDINATING LUNGE OPENER

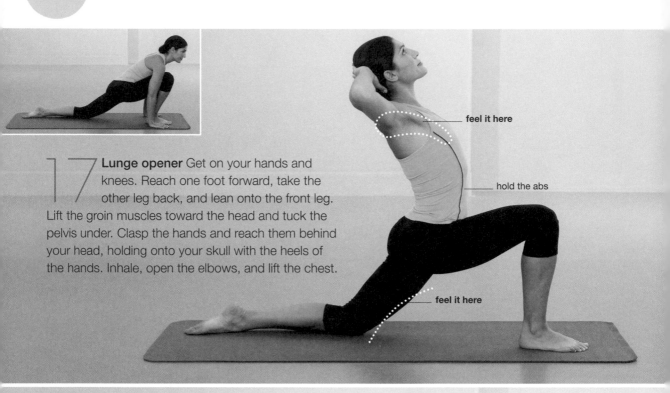

17 **Lunge opener** Get on your hands and knees. Reach one foot forward, take the other leg back, and lean onto the front leg. Lift the groin muscles toward the head and tuck the pelvis under. Clasp the hands and reach them behind your head, holding onto your skull with the heels of the hands. Inhale, open the elbows, and lift the chest.

feel it here

hold the abs

feel it here

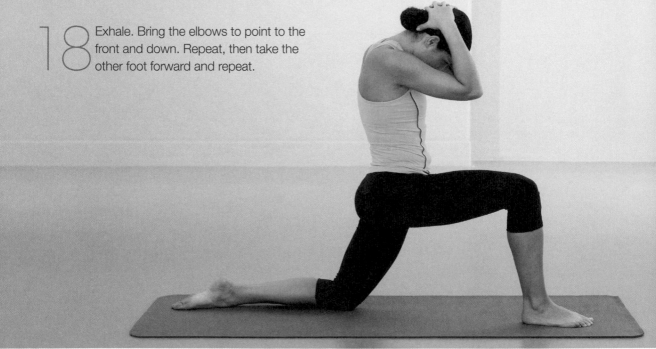

18 Exhale. Bring the elbows to point to the front and down. Repeat, then take the other foot forward and repeat.

LIMBERING ROUND BACK SQUAT

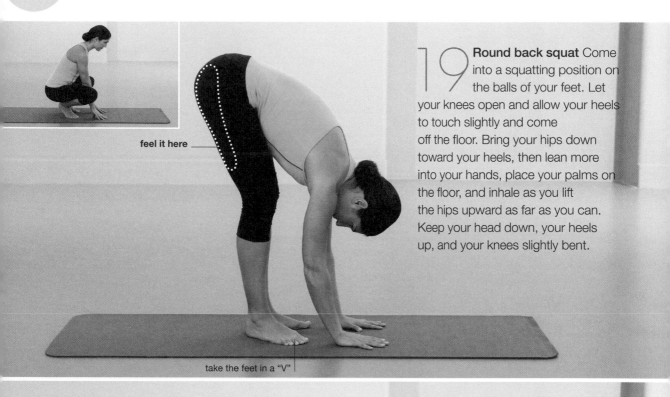

feel it here

take the feet in a "V"

19 **Round back squat** Come into a squatting position on the balls of your feet. Let your knees open and allow your heels to touch slightly and come off the floor. Bring your hips down toward your heels, then lean more into your hands, place your palms on the floor, and inhale as you lift the hips upward as far as you can. Keep your head down, your heels up, and your knees slightly bent.

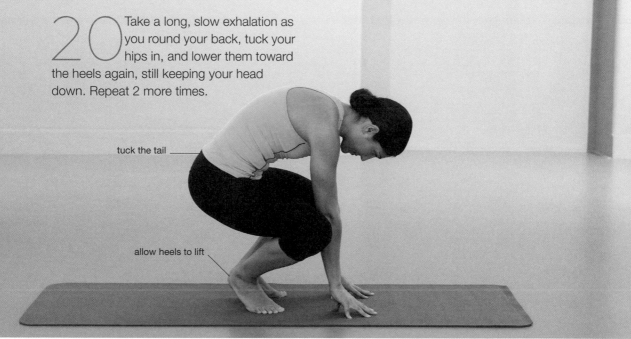

20 Take a long, slow exhalation as you round your back, tuck your hips in, and lower them toward the heels again, still keeping your head down. Repeat 2 more times.

tuck the tail

allow heels to lift

ELONGATING HANGING STRETCH

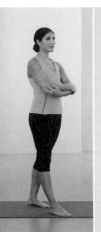

21 **Hanging stretch**
Roll up to standing and place one foot ahead of the other, about your foot's distance and a hand-width apart. Hold onto something if you cannot keep your balance; otherwise fold your arms in front of you and hold onto your elbows. Firm the hips and pull your navel to your spine (see p17). Inhale, then tuck your chin under and round your upper back, allowing your head to hang.

22 Exhale, scoop deeper into your spine, and lower your head to hip-height as if you were going over an imaginary fence. Repeat 2 more times, then change legs and repeat on the other side.

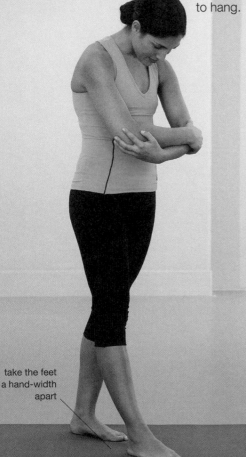

take the feet a hand-width apart

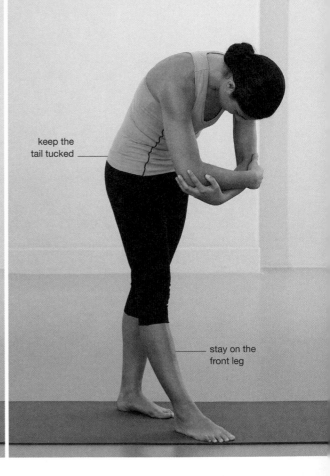

keep the tail tucked

stay on the front leg

CENTERING TOP-TO-TOE STRETCH

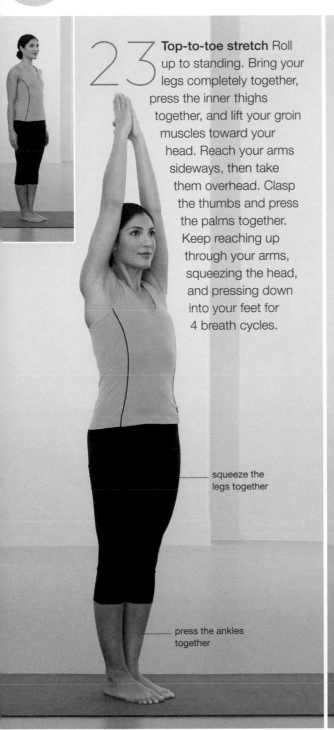

23 **Top-to-toe stretch** Roll up to standing. Bring your legs completely together, press the inner thighs together, and lift your groin muscles toward your head. Reach your arms sideways, then take them overhead. Clasp the thumbs and press the palms together. Keep reaching up through your arms, squeezing the head, and pressing down into your feet for 4 breath cycles.

squeeze the legs together

press the ankles together

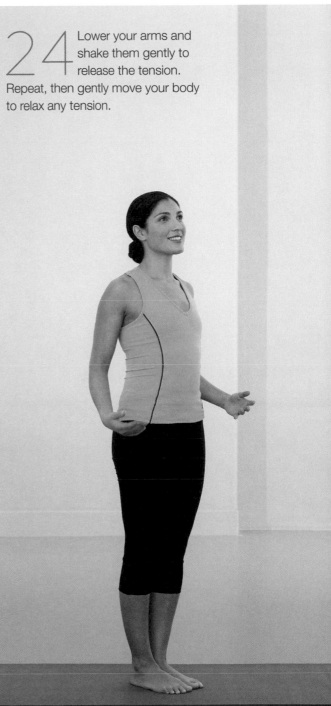

24 Lower your arms and shake them gently to release the tension. Repeat, then gently move your body to relax any tension.

POSTURE STRETCH AT A GLANCE

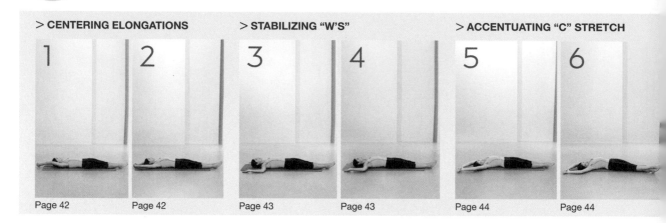

> CENTERING ELONGATIONS

1
Page 42

2
Page 42

> STABILIZING "W'S"

3
Page 43

4
Page 43

> ACCENTUATING "C" STRETCH

5
Page 44

6
Page 44

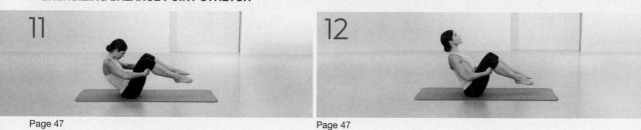

> ENERGIZING BALANCE POINT STRETCH

11
Page 47

12
Page 47

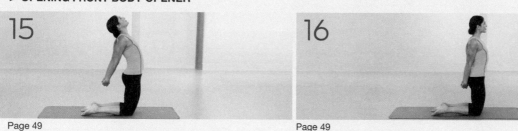

> OPENING FRONT BODY OPENER

15
Page 49

16
Page 49

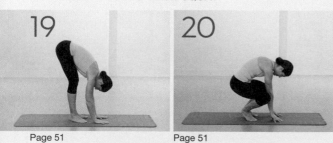

> LIMBERING ROUND BACK SQUAT

19
Page 51

20
Page 51

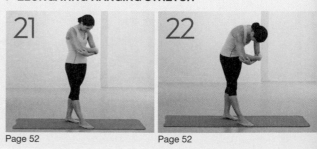

> ELONGATING HANGING STRETCH

21
Page 52

22
Page 52

> SOFTENING BABY ROCKS

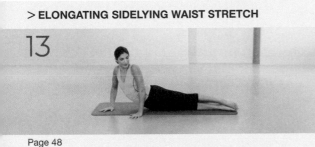

7 — Page 45

8 — Page 45

> ARTICULATING HURDLER LAT STRETCH

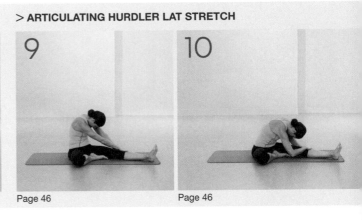

9 — Page 46

10 — Page 46

> ELONGATING SIDELYING WAIST STRETCH

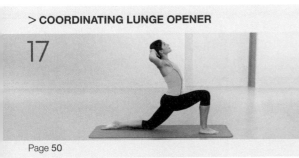

13 — Page 48

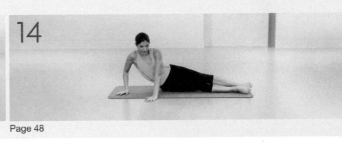

14 — Page 48

> COORDINATING LUNGE OPENER

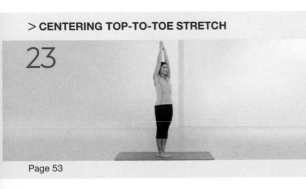

17 — Page 50

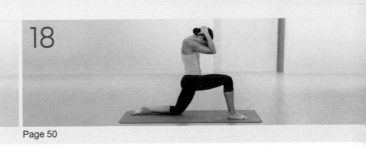

18 — Page 50

> CENTERING TOP-TO-TOE STRETCH

23 — Page 53

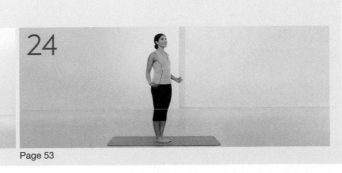

24 — Page 53

POSTURE STRETCH FAQS

The difference is in the details when it comes to developing and maintaining good posture. Take these tips to heart. Examine yourself in a mirror and learn to see the subtle nuances that cumulatively add up to a vibrant posture. After a while, you're sure to see the changes.

WHAT EXACTLY IS GOING ON IN MY BODY IN THE ELONGATIONS?

Although seemingly simple, the Elongations begin to stretch out every molecule of your body. Think of your body volumetrically, three-dimensionally. Imagine your torso is a cylinder, whose front is much more pliable than the back. Tightening the front helps to stretch out the tighter parts at the back. Elongating the whole body is just like stretching out a long roll of clay, but you have to soften the clay before you can stretch it.

MY HEAD AND ARMS DON'T TOUCH THE FLOOR IN THE "W'S." WHAT SHOULD I DO?

Not to worry. Fold a towel and place it under your head. Then place pillows under each arm. It's common for people to start slightly off the floor in the "W's," partly because we rarely lie completely flat in bed at night. I often push away the pillows when I awaken, and then do my "W's" to start the day. It combats the contorted positions we sometimes assume during sleep.

THE "C" STRETCH SEEMS HARD TO DO. HOW CAN I TELL I'M DOING IT CORRECTLY?

Move the upper part of your body first. Then add the lower body. Be sure to feel the entire length of the "C," from the wrist all the way to the ankle. The "C" is so beneficial because it addresses the sides of the body, which are often neglected in more general stretching. Especially when working to achieve postural change, side stretches of the upper rib cage, armpit, waist, and the sides of the legs are necessary to acquire a straighter standing position, and to balance the right side of the body in relation to the left.

THE SIDELYING WAIST STRETCH IS HARD TO FEEL. HOW CAN I INTENSIFY IT?

Make sure you are lifting your groin muscles strongly toward your head. Press your hips forward. The side of the body nearest the floor is again making a long "C" shape. So work to make it as long as possible, reaching your bottom foot away from the ear on the same side. Increase the top curve of the "C" by lifting your uppermost ear toward the ceiling. Use the hands to twist your hips in relation to the shoulders.

WHAT DO I DO IF I CAN'T STRAIGHTEN OUT MY HIPS IN THE FRONT BODY OPENER?

Don't panic. There's always another way. Kneel on padding if your knees are too sensitive. Usually a mat or folded towel works best. Sometimes pillows are worse because the knees dig into them. Next, squeeze your buttock cheeks together and tighten your glutes, to stretch the front of the hips. Still need help? Balance by holding onto a piece of furniture, press down on your hands, and lift your chest.

HOW DO I DO THE HANGING STRETCH IF MY BACK FEELS AS IF IT'S MOVING IN CHUNKS?

This is a common issue for many people when they start to work with their spine. Think of the spine as being like a child's wooden segmented toy snake. The chunks you feel are groups of those segments moving together, instead of individually. Try to keep thinking about rolling over an imaginary fence and keep imagining the individual parts of the spine moving in turn—the neck, the upper back, the middle back.

WHAT MUST I FOCUS ON IN KNEELING STRETCHES? ALL I CAN THINK ABOUT IS THE PRESSURE ON MY KNEES.

First of all, use padding if you feel any discomfort, then you can concentrate on finding your smile lines (see p16). Try to press the hips forward and press each knee equally into the floor. This is a great position for gaining low-back strength, and to help out any problems with leg length.

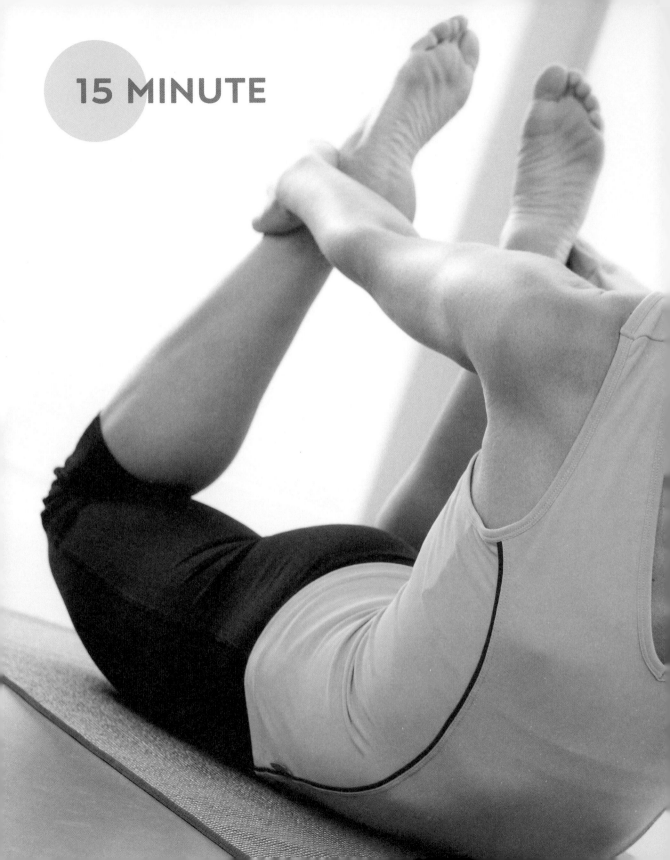

15 MINUTE

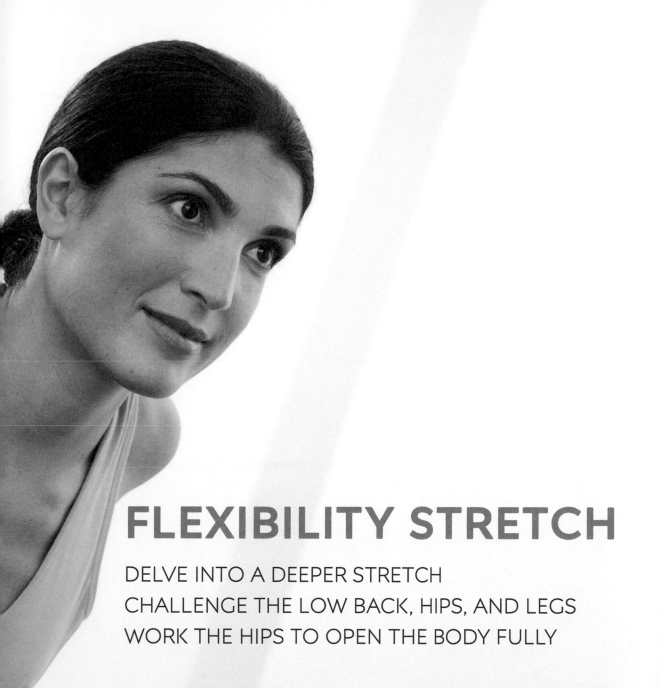

FLEXIBILITY STRETCH

DELVE INTO A DEEPER STRETCH
CHALLENGE THE LOW BACK, HIPS, AND LEGS
WORK THE HIPS TO OPEN THE BODY FULLY

FLEXIBILITY STRETCH

Flexibility is best understood as developing your own potential. Each body is unique, with its own set of bone shapes and muscle lengths. Take the challenge here to continue opening your entire body through the gateway of the hips. Hip suppleness is essential to spinal health.

The best way to achieve full-body flexibility is to take on the challenge of the low back, hips, and legs. Many people give up when they feel they are not flexible in the hamstrings, but remember that the body also comprises fascial tissue (see p10) that, among other roles, ties the biomechanics of the upper body to that of the lower body. Now that you've done some loosening and lengthening of your whole body, it's time to focus on a deeper opening of your lower body. This sequence offers more moves that combine stretches with circular, rotational movements. It may require more modification than the first two workouts. Have heart. Challenging yourself with many different exercises will help you identify your weak areas. There is always a back door to a movement—a way in which you can break it down and simply perform parts of it until they transform into old, familiar friends. Then you can join them together again and you're there!

THE EXERCISES

The Knee Pumps prepare the legs and hips for the next moves. Part of my daily ritual, Knee Pumps help keep my knees and sciatic nerves—the long nerve along the backs of the legs—supple. There is no harm, and it is very beneficial, if you take the extra time to increase the repetitions to as many as 20 on each leg.

The Quad Stretch, Thigh Sweep, Fouetté Stretch, and Figure 4 Stretch are absolutely essential to my personal regimen. Go slow at first and take care to observe the transitions from one movement to the

> ### TIPS FOR FLEXIBILITY STRETCH
>
> - **Suspend judgment** about your hip and leg stretch. Slow, steady persistence pays off. Look to yourself, and in yourself, for comparison.
>
> - **Be sure to energize** your upper body as well as your lower body to create the necessary full-body connection.
>
> - **Always use straps**, belts, or bands to modify when needed.
>
> - **Changing the length of tight**, stiff muscles takes time. If your body type is overly flexible, tighten yourself and make the motion or position smaller so as not to over-stretch.

next. Work hard to make these transitions smooth; they are actually additional stretches that help give the sequence its three-dimensional element.

Challenge yourself to master the sequence by imagining you are coaching someone and have to demonstrate and explain each move to them. Being a teacher forces you to think about the nature of each movement and is the best way to clarify them in your own mind.

When you get to the Lying Hamstring Stretch and Advancing Frogs, work hard to coordinate all the various parts. It may seem overwhelming to think of them all at once, so first start with the obvious—

the basic shape. Again, modify, modify, modify.
Rome wasn't built in a day. The next two moves, the
Straddle and the Pull-the-thread Lunge give
you a bit of a rest.

Try the Angel Flight Stretch. Remember, your
shape and range will be different than the model's,
so start low and slow. This stretch is the ultimate in
opening the entire front of the pelvis and thighs. Stick
with it, and I promise that you will transform beyond
all of your expectations.

The Cobbler Stretch is the gateway to opening the stretch of
the hips. In this position, it is important to respect the "voice" of
the knees and not over-stretch.

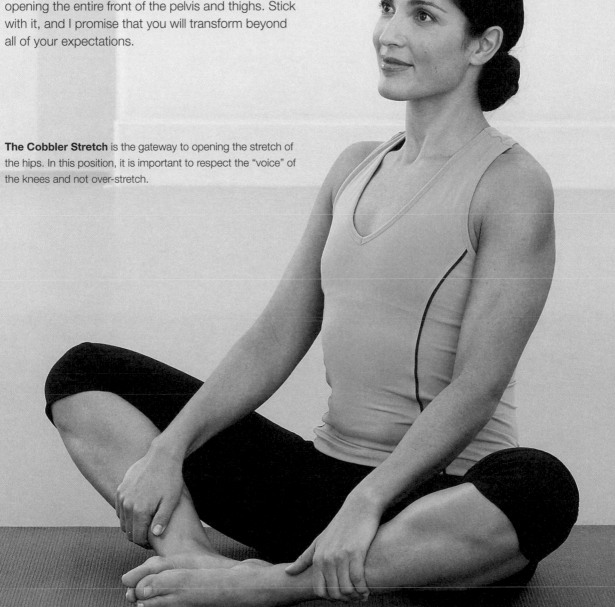

LIMBERING KNEE PUMPS

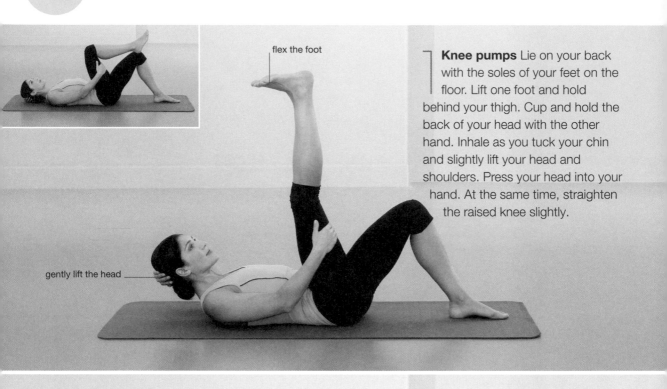

flex the foot

gently lift the head

1 **Knee pumps** Lie on your back with the soles of your feet on the floor. Lift one foot and hold behind your thigh. Cup and hold the back of your head with the other hand. Inhale as you tuck your chin and slightly lift your head and shoulders. Press your head into your hand. At the same time, straighten the raised knee slightly.

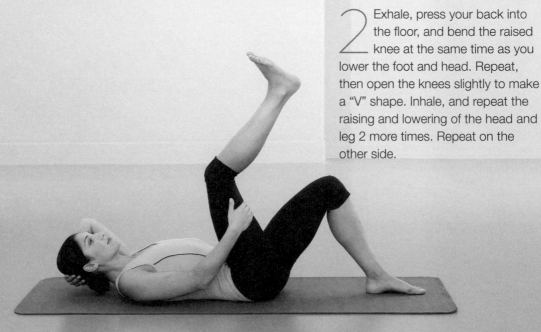

2 Exhale, press your back into the floor, and bend the raised knee at the same time as you lower the foot and head. Repeat, then open the knees slightly to make a "V" shape. Inhale, and repeat the raising and lowering of the head and leg 2 more times. Repeat on the other side.

ENERGIZING BABY ROLLS

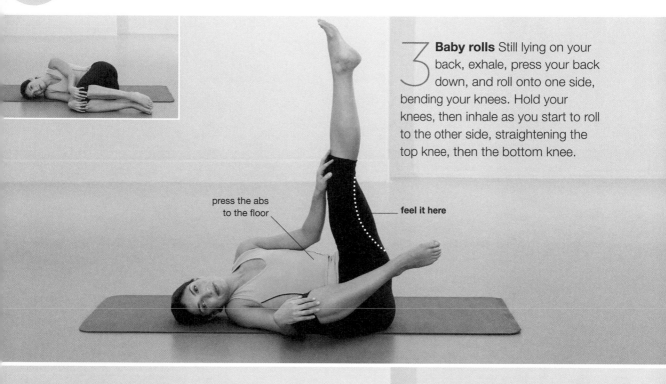

3 **Baby rolls** Still lying on your back, exhale, press your back down, and roll onto one side, bending your knees. Hold your knees, then inhale as you start to roll to the other side, straightening the top knee, then the bottom knee.

press the abs to the floor

feel it here

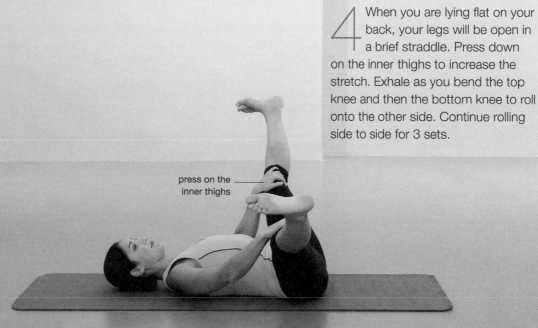

4 When you are lying flat on your back, your legs will be open in a brief straddle. Press down on the inner thighs to increase the stretch. Exhale as you bend the top knee and then the bottom knee to roll onto the other side. Continue rolling side to side for 3 sets.

press on the inner thighs

ELONGATING COBBLER STRETCH

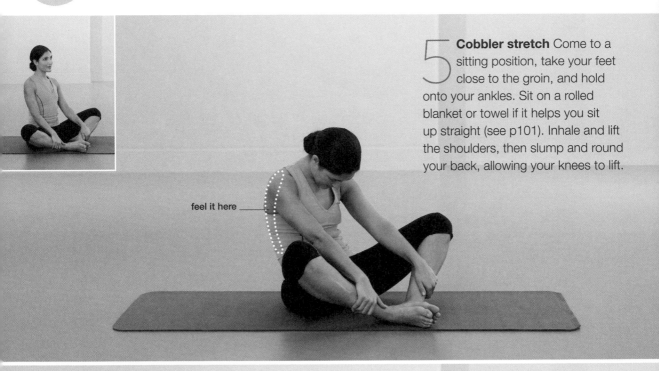

5 **Cobbler stretch** Come to a sitting position, take your feet close to the groin, and hold onto your ankles. Sit on a rolled blanket or towel if it helps you sit up straight (see p101). Inhale and lift the shoulders, then slump and round your back, allowing your knees to lift.

feel it here

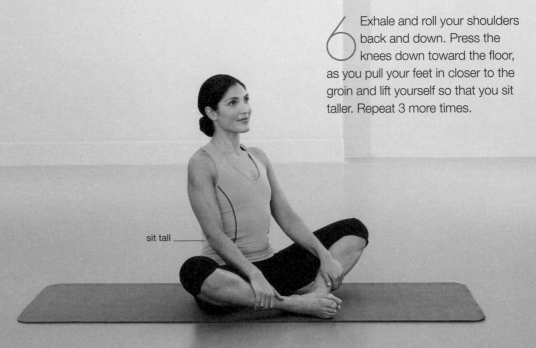

6 Exhale and roll your shoulders back and down. Press the knees down toward the floor, as you pull your feet in closer to the groin and lift yourself so that you sit taller. Repeat 3 more times.

sit tall

ARTICULATING QUAD STRETCH

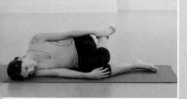

7 **Quad stretch** Lie on your side and bend both knees up toward your chest. Hold onto your bottom knee. Use a pillow under your neck if you feel any strain (see p101). Inhale, hold onto your top ankle, and pull your top knee gently toward your chest.

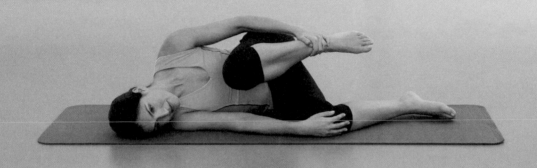

8 Exhale, then smoothly pull your top knee back. Do not let the bottom knee be pulled backward by the top leg. Stay, then pull backward a little more on the top knee. Repeat. Release your ankle and go onto your back, then return to your side and straighten your legs.

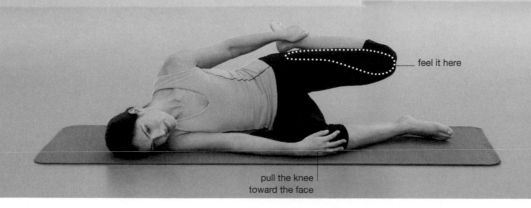

feel it here

pull the knee toward the face

ELONGATING THIGH SWEEP

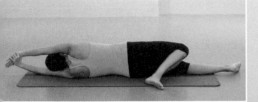

9 **Thigh sweep** Take your arms overhead on the floor and bend your top knee backward. Hold the wrist on the side of the bent leg, then inhale and slowly pull your wrist out and beyond your head as you roll backward toward the floor. Do not force it, and remember to modify the position of the knee if you find it uncomfortable.

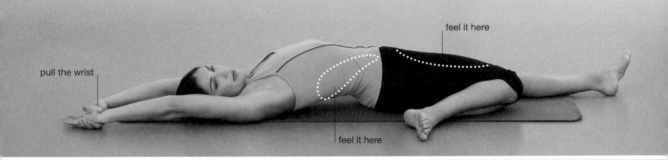

feel it here

pull the wrist

feel it here

10 Exhale, tuck your pelvis under, pull your wrist again, and roll to face forward toward the floor. Repeat, inhaling as you roll backward and exhaling as you roll forward.

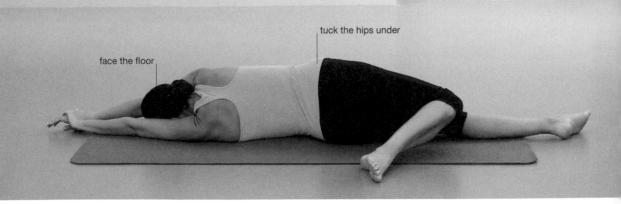

tuck the hips under

face the floor

STIMULATING FOUETTÉ STRETCH

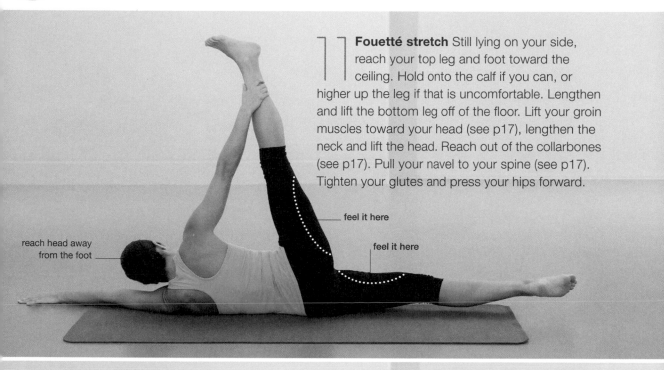

11 Fouetté stretch Still lying on your side, reach your top leg and foot toward the ceiling. Hold onto the calf if you can, or higher up the leg if that is uncomfortable. Lengthen and lift the bottom leg off of the floor. Lift your groin muscles toward your head (see p17), lengthen the neck and lift the head. Reach out of the collarbones (see p17). Pull your navel to your spine (see p17). Tighten your glutes and press your hips forward.

feel it here

feel it here

reach head away from the foot

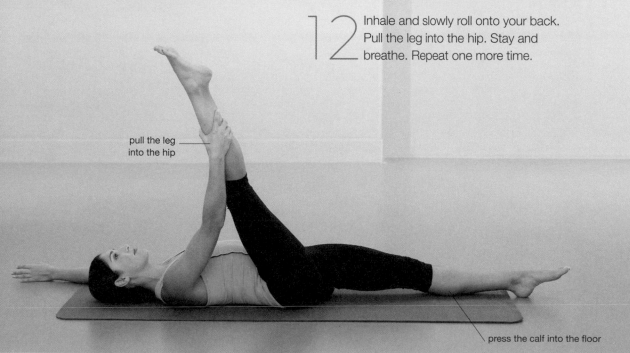

12 Inhale and slowly roll onto your back. Pull the leg into the hip. Stay and breathe. Repeat one more time.

pull the leg into the hip

press the calf into the floor

BALANCING FIGURE 4 STRETCH

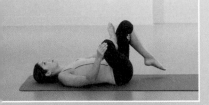

13 **Figure 4 stretch** Go onto your back, bend your knees, and place one ankle on the other thigh. Place one hand underneath that thigh and the palm of the other hand on the knee of the crossed leg. Lift the groin muscles toward the head to stabilize the spine. Inhale and pull the hand behind the thigh toward your chest.

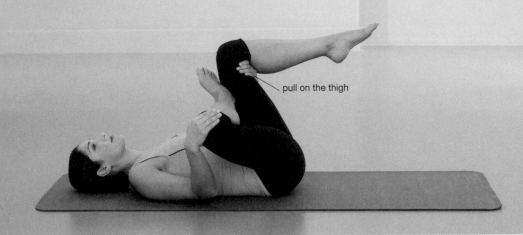

pull on the thigh

14 Exhale and press the hand against the knee, away from your face, keeping the bent leg parallel to the floor. If the knee hurts, come out of the position, or loosen the posture. Repeat. Release both legs, thump your thighs, and breathe normally. Roll onto the other side and repeat Steps 7 to 14.

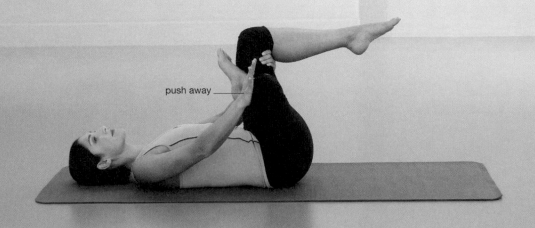

push away

COORDINATING LYING HAMSTRING STRETCH

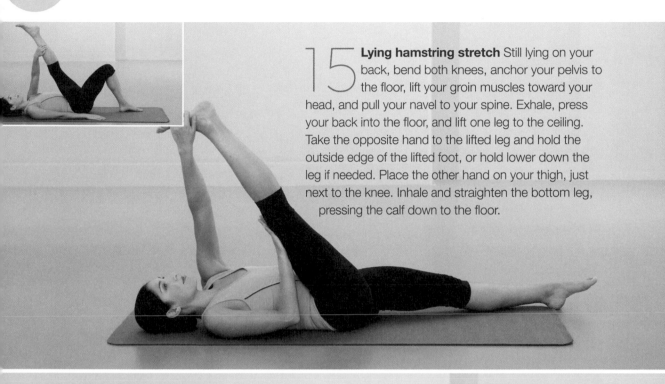

15 **Lying hamstring stretch** Still lying on your back, bend both knees, anchor your pelvis to the floor, lift your groin muscles toward your head, and pull your navel to your spine. Exhale, press your back into the floor, and lift one leg to the ceiling. Take the opposite hand to the lifted leg and hold the outside edge of the lifted foot, or hold lower down the leg if needed. Place the other hand on your thigh, just next to the knee. Inhale and straighten the bottom leg, pressing the calf down to the floor.

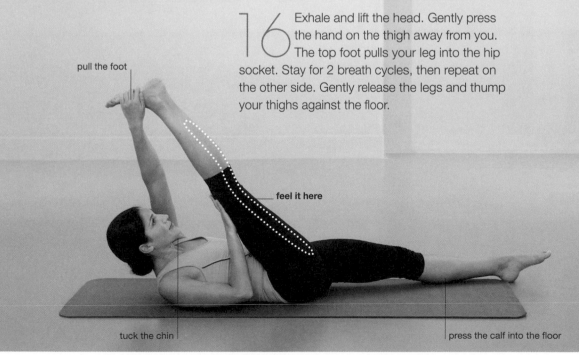

16 Exhale and lift the head. Gently press the hand on the thigh away from you. The top foot pulls your leg into the hip socket. Stay for 2 breath cycles, then repeat on the other side. Gently release the legs and thump your thighs against the floor.

pull the foot

feel it here

tuck the chin

press the calf into the floor

17 **Advancing frogs** Come onto your hands and knees, open your knees, reach your arms forward, and squat back, bringing your hips close to your heels. Support your back by lifting the abs. Stay for 2 breath cycles.

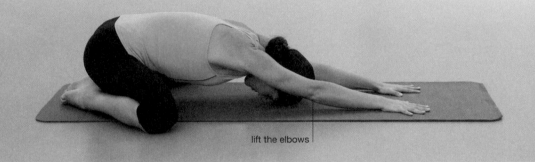

lift the elbows

18 Move your torso and arms forward, and come up on your forearms. Actively press the inner edges of your heels into the floor. Your heels will come apart. Lift the groin muscles toward the head to avoid slumping in the low back. Stay for 2 breath cycles.

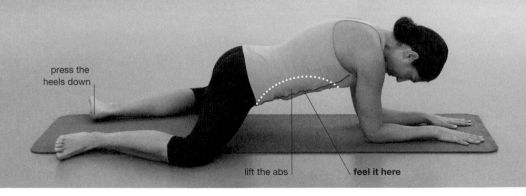

press the heels down

lift the abs

feel it here

LENGTHENING STRADDLE

19 **Straddle** Come to a sitting position, sitting evenly on your sitbones, with your legs open to at least a 90° angle, and with your toes pulled toward your head. Lift your back and open your chest. Sit on a rolled blanket or towel if it helps you to sit up straight, or bend your knees. Lift the groin muscles up toward the head. Open your arms strongly sideways and reach out through the head, legs, and arms.

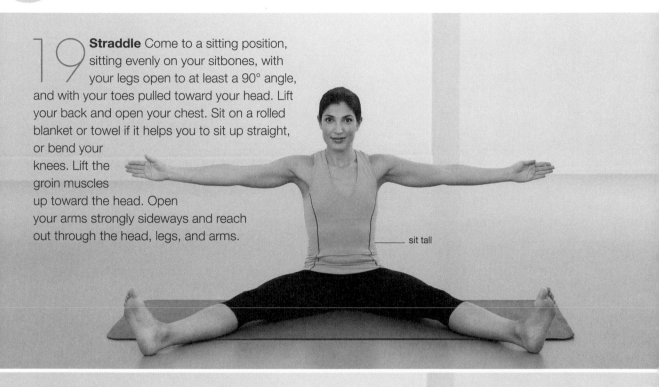

sit tall

20 Inhale and reach up and over an imaginary fence to one side. Rest the lower hand on the floor behind the outstretched leg. Firm your waist. Exhale, then return to center by "painting the ceiling" with your top arm. Repeat on the other side, then release. Gently roll your shoulders to relax.

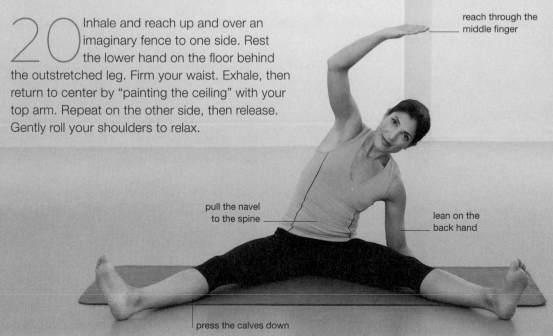

reach through the middle finger

pull the navel to the spine

lean on the back hand

press the calves down

STABILIZING PULL-THE-THREAD LUNGE

22 **Pull-the-thread lunge** Go onto your hands and knees, take one leg in front, and lean into it, palms on either side of the front foot. Line up the bent-leg knee and toes straight ahead in front of the hip. Press the foot into the floor. Extend the other leg straight behind you and tuck the pelvis under strongly.

tuck the tail under

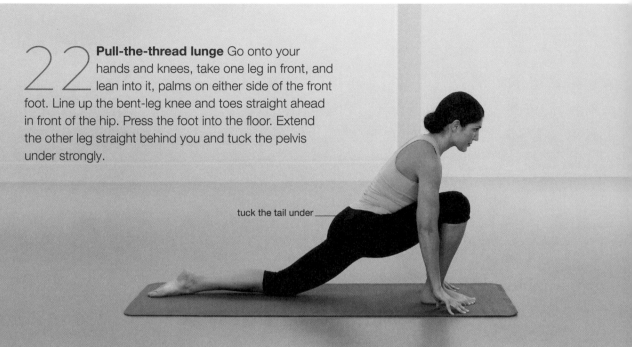

22 Pull an imaginary thread up to the ceiling with the hand on the side of the extended leg. Look up at the hand and press down into the floor with the other hand. Stay for 2 breath cycles. Take the hand down to the floor, then repeat with the other leg in front.

look at the "thread"

tighten the waist

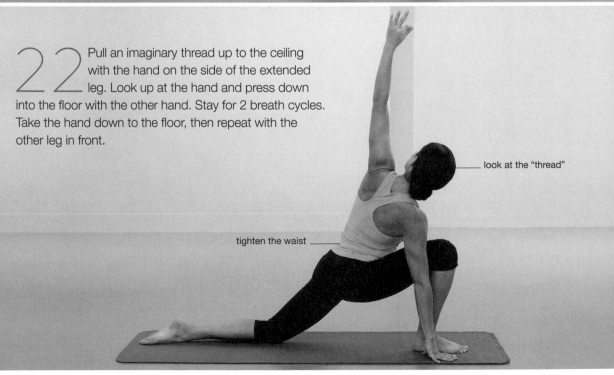

POWERING ANGEL FLIGHT STRETCH

23 **Angel flight stretch** Lie on your stomach, face turned to one side. Feel the imaginary swimming-pool water lifting your abdomen off the floor (see p16). Press the tailbone down toward the heels. Inhale, then reach back and bend the knees to hold onto your ankles.

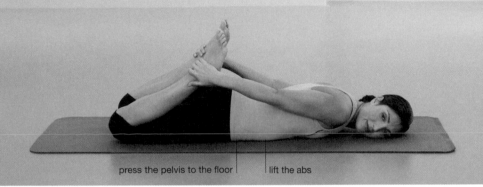

press the pelvis to the floor   lift the abs

24 Exhale, press your feet against your hands, and lift your chest and thighs off the floor to make a bowlike shape. Stay for 2 breath cycles, then release your hands and feet and relax for another 2 breath cycles, breathing deeply.

press the feet against the hands

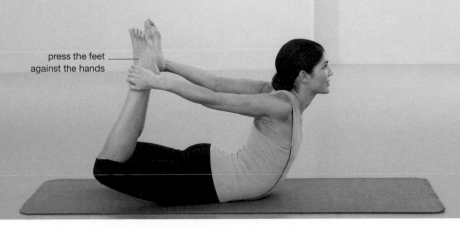

FLEXIBILITY STRETCH AT A GLANCE

> LIMBERING KNEE PUMPS

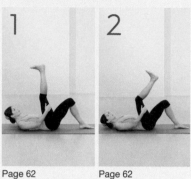

1

Page 62

2

Page 62

> ENERGIZING BABY ROLLS

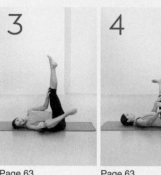

3

Page 63

4

Page 63

> ELONGATING COBBLER STRETCH

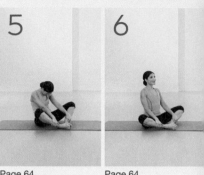

5

Page 64

6

Page 64

> STIMULATING FOUETTÉ STRETCH

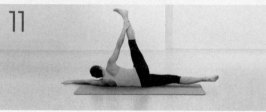

11

Page 67

12

Page 67

> COORDINATING LYING HAMSTRING STRETCH

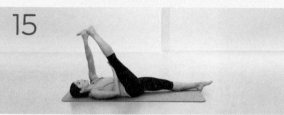

15

Page 69

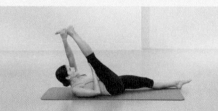

16

Page 69

> LENGTHENING STRADDLE

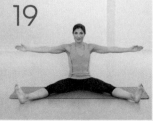

19

Page 71

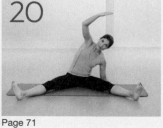

20

Page 71

> STABILIZING PULL-THE-THREAD LUNGE

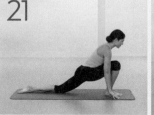

21

Page 72

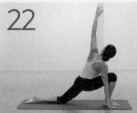

22

Page 72

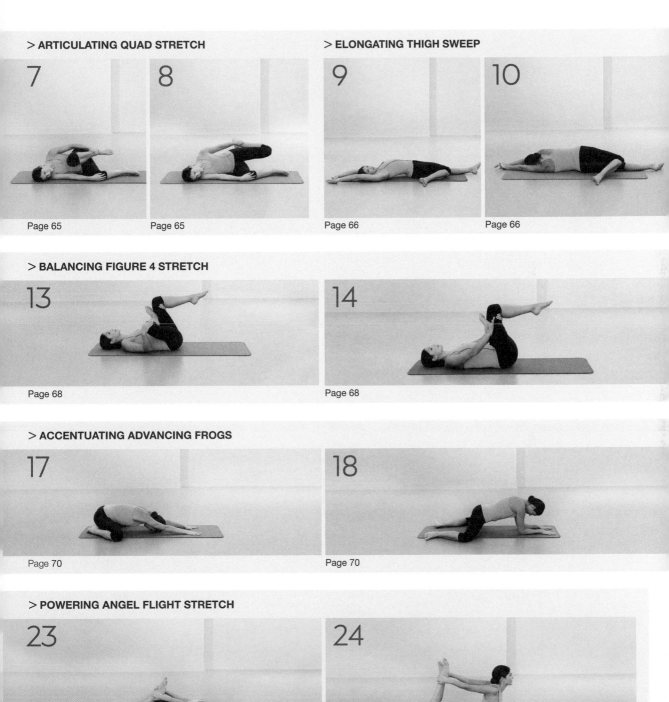

> ARTICULATING QUAD STRETCH

7

Page 65

8

Page 65

> ELONGATING THIGH SWEEP

9

Page 66

10

Page 66

> BALANCING FIGURE 4 STRETCH

13

Page 68

14

Page 68

> ACCENTUATING ADVANCING FROGS

17

Page 70

18

Page 70

> POWERING ANGEL FLIGHT STRETCH

23

Page 73

24

Page 73

FLEXIBILITY STRETCH FAQS

This program begins the true challenge to developing your potential to stretch, so take extra care not to force or strain. Here are some common questions and tips about how to modify positions that seem impossible and how to direct the stretch into the proper location for the best effect.

WHAT DO THE KNEE PUMPS STRETCH?

The Knee Pumps stretch many parts of the hips and legs. The inner thigh and hamstring muscles are the most obvious. Not so obvious are the sciatic nerves, the big nerves that run from the pelvis into the legs. Adding the head lifts to the knee movements adds even more stretch. Combining different body parts in one exercise helps stretch the fascia, the connective bands that hold the body structures together as though they were wrapped in plastic wrap (see pp10–11).

WHY DO I HAVE TO HOLD ONTO THE BOTTOM KNEE IN THE QUAD STRETCH?

Holding the bottom knee ensures that the stretch is being directed into the front of the hip joint and not into the waistline. It may seem awkward at first, but with time it will become natural. Work hard to find the line between the buttocks and the hamstrings as you pull the foot backward. This will help you gain the best possible stretch of the front of the dense thigh.

WHAT DO I DO IF MY KNEE HURTS IN THE THIGH SWEEP?

Always make sure your knee is not over-stretching in any of the stretches. You should never feel pain directly in the knee. If it does hurt, you can simply straighten the leg on top, open your legs slightly, and brace them against the floor. Then, tighten your hips and press them forward as you pull on the wrist, turning the chest forward and back.

WHAT DOES "FOUETTÉ" MEAN, AND WHAT DOES THIS EXERCISE ACHIEVE?

It means "whipped" and the action is easy to see when a ballet dancer performs a fouetté. The movement gives a three-dimensional stretch deep inside your hip. You have to imagine the internal roundness of the hip joint, the way the head of the thigh bone moves in the socket of the pelvis. The circular movement created by the Fouetté Stretch improves the mobility of that joint and of your entire pelvis.

IS IT NECESSARY FOR ME TO HOLD THE OUTSIDE OF THE OPPOSITE FOOT IN THE LYING HAMSTRING STRETCH? I CAN'T REACH IT.

This is an instance where having a stretching strap can come in handy. A bathrobe belt also works well. Loop the belt around your foot and hold it with the hand on the opposite side. Press the other hand against the thigh of the lifted leg, even if you cannot straighten the leg. You have to start somewhere. You can and will improve.

I CAN'T EVEN REMOTELY BEGIN TO GET INTO THE ANGEL FLIGHT STRETCH. CAN YOU HELP?

This is a challenging exercise, even for veteran stretchers. Again, the use of a belt can help here. You can even start by holding one leg, then the other since there are two repetitions of the exercise. An alternative is to lie on your stomach on the floor with your feet behind you over a sofa seat. Then press your hands against the floor and lift your chest as in the Modified Cobra (see p32).

I ONLY FEEL PRESSURE IN MY KNEES IN ADVANCING FROGS. WHERE SHOULD I FEEL THE STRETCH?

First, try to get your knees as open as possible and place the weight on the inside of the knees, not on top of the kneecaps. You should feel the stretch deep in the innermost fold of the leg at the groin. Be sure to keep the waist lifted since that takes pressure off the inner thigh. Use your hands and forearms to direct the pressure back and down toward the inner thigh.

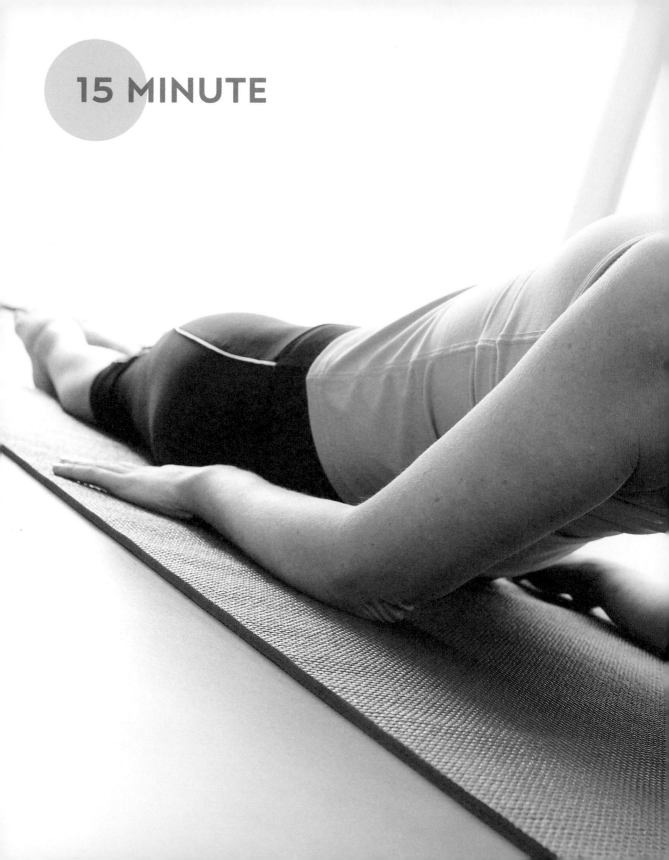

15 MINUTE

STRENGTH STRETCH

FIND YOUR PEAK OF PERFORMANCE
BE STRONG YET LITHE
FLUIDITY LEADS TO EASE AND GRACE

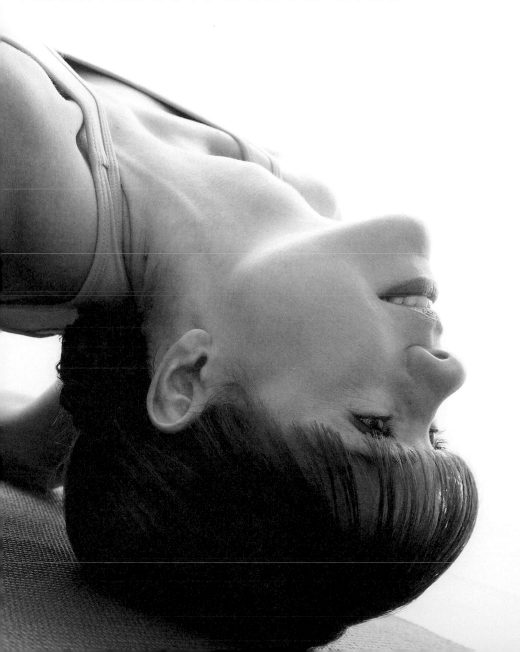

STRENGTH STRETCH

You don't need to be a contortionist to master this final sequence. Use your body control to guide you into these more advanced movements. Regard it as your ultimate goal. Even beginners can discover how much control they need to exert, whether they are trying to balance in a precarious pose or performing the simplest stretch.

Strength by definition means grounding and control. See this sequence as one feat of strength after another in an Olympic trial. Close up, one can see the suppleness of the athlete's body, and in action you can see the litheness of their motions. Think of all the hours of preparation Olympic athletes must endure to reach their final goal. In this sequence, look at each exercise as a goal in and of itself. The trick is to break each exercise down by starting small and gradually building to a larger and steadier range of motion. Remember that achieving a general level of fitness takes about two months of practice, and developing a split may take more like six months, depending on how naturally flexible you are. The recipe for Olympic development is to stress the body, then to rest it. Be smart and give your body a good rest after practicing this sequence. The poses and movements here move toward a crescendo that primes you for success.

THE EXERCISES

Set the tone for strength by standing tall in the Butterfly Stretch and the Upper Side Bend. Feel your upper body moving against the lower body, as if your lower body were rooted and anchored, like a great oak tree. The series of squats that follows coordinates the strength and suppleness of the spine with the suppleness of the legs. Get more benefit by opening your knees as wide as you can in the Wide Squat Twist and in the Deep Squat. These

squats also provide a great opportunity to strengthen the "pelvic diaphragm"—the parachutelike muscle layer that lies at the bottom of the torso.

As you perform the next exercise, the Neck Stretch, be mindful that you are now coordinating the "neck diaphragm"—the parachutelike muscle and soft tissue layers defining the top of the rib cage—with the pelvic diaphragm. So this sequence works on more than meets the eye. It is the ultimate in strength and control. Become willing to acquire the ability to coordinate deep muscles with the larger, more obvious muscles, such as the abs, the glutes, and the thighs.

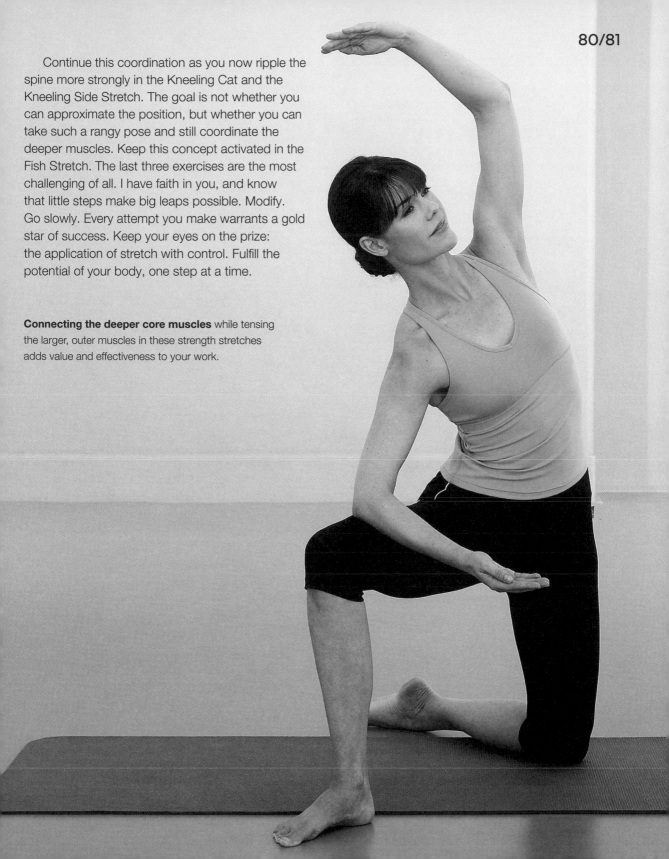

Continue this coordination as you now ripple the spine more strongly in the Kneeling Cat and the Kneeling Side Stretch. The goal is not whether you can approximate the position, but whether you can take such a rangy pose and still coordinate the deeper muscles. Keep this concept activated in the Fish Stretch. The last three exercises are the most challenging of all. I have faith in you, and know that little steps make big leaps possible. Modify. Go slowly. Every attempt you make warrants a gold star of success. Keep your eyes on the prize: the application of stretch with control. Fulfill the potential of your body, one step at a time.

Connecting the deeper core muscles while tensing the larger, outer muscles in these strength stretches adds value and effectiveness to your work.

LIMBERING BUTTERFLY STRETCH

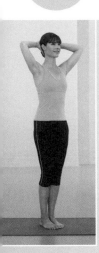

1 **Butterfly stretch** Stand with legs completely together and pressing the base of the big and little toes, and the middle of the heel of both feet on the floor. Lift your groin muscles toward the head (see p17). Pull your navel to your spine (see p17). Clasp your hands behind your head, inhale, and lift up and forward from your waist. Simultaneously bow your head, bend your knees, and bring the elbows toward each other.

2 Exhale, straighten the legs, and stretch up and out of your waist, fanning the elbows open. Reach out through the points of the elbows and feel as if your breastbone is being pulled up toward the ceiling. Repeat, then relax and shake the hands.

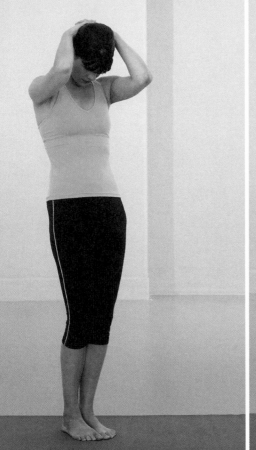

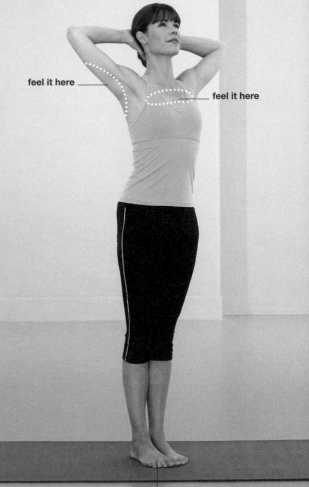

feel it here

feel it here

anchor the feet

OPENING UPPER SIDE BEND

3 **Upper side bend** Still with your legs completely together, renew your form. Lift the groin muscles toward the head, and pull the abs up and into your spine. Clasp your hands behind your head.

4 Inhale and lift up and out of the rib cage, over an imaginary fence under one armpit. Tilt one elbow down toward the floor, the other up toward the ceiling. Exhale and take your shoulders back to center. Feel a "V" of strength from the small of the low back to the points of the elbows. Repeat on the other side, and then repeat one more set.

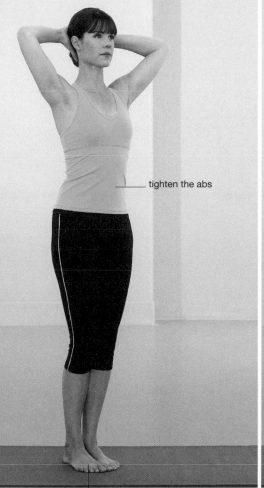

tighten the abs

anchor the feet

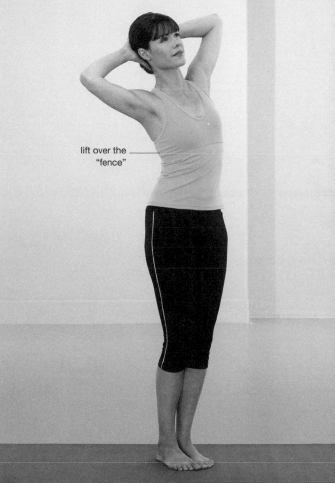

lift over the "fence"

LENGTHENING FLAT BACK SQUAT

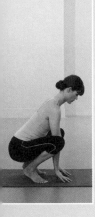

5 **Flat back squat** Lift the abs and roll down your spine into a squatting position. Let your knees open and go onto the balls of your feet. Lean on your hands, then inhale as you lift diagonally up and out with your chest, keeping your back flat and extended. Imagine you are looking under a table.

6 Exhale slowly as you lift the hips upward, taking the heels as high as you can. Straighten your knees and tuck your chin into the legs. Keep lifting the groin muscles toward the head. Stay and breathe, then repeat, intensifying the stretch at the end. Lower and relax. Repeat.

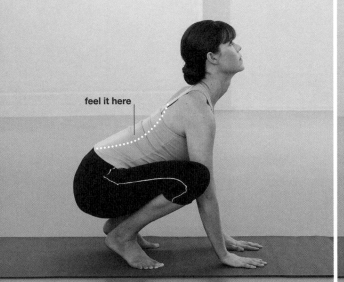

feel it here

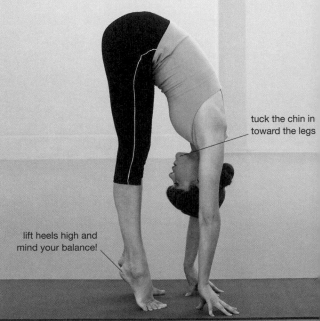

tuck the chin in toward the legs

lift heels high and mind your balance!

STIMULATING WIDE SQUAT TWIST

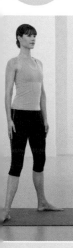

7 **Wide squat twist** Come to a standing position with your feet wider than hip-width apart and your toes facing outward. Lift the groin muscles toward the head, inhale, and lower your hips. Bring your hands to the thighs, take some of your weight into them, and check that your toes are in line with your knees.

8 Inhale, then press backward on one hand on the inside of the knee, twisting that shoulder down. Look up and out in the opposite direction. Stay for 2 breath cycles, then exhale and bring the shoulders back to center. Come up, shake your legs a little, and repeat on the other side.

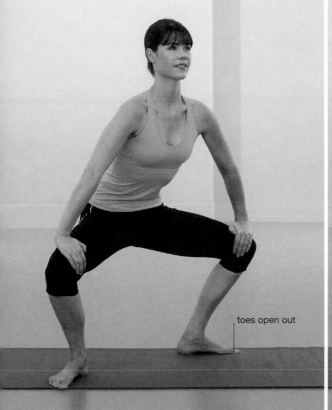

toes open out

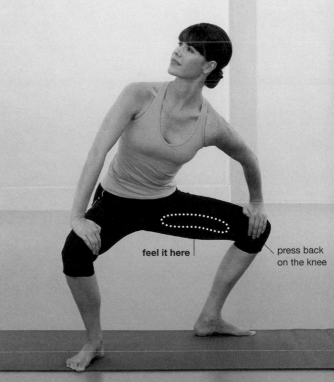

feel it here

press back on the knee

SUSTAINING DEEP SQUAT

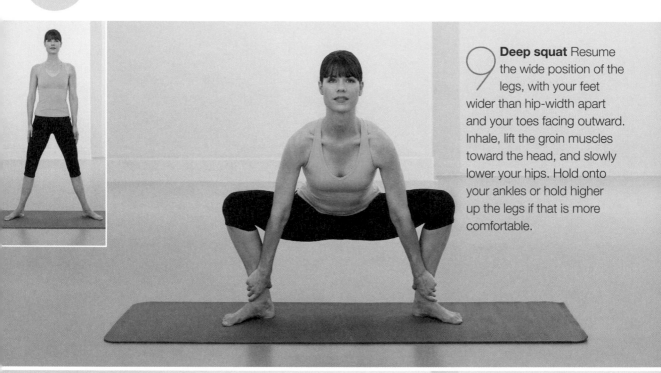

9 **Deep squat** Resume the wide position of the legs, with your feet wider than hip-width apart and your toes facing outward. Inhale, lift the groin muscles toward the head, and slowly lower your hips. Hold onto your ankles or hold higher up the legs if that is more comfortable.

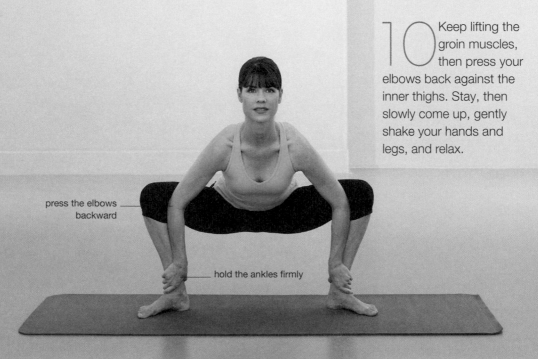

10 Keep lifting the groin muscles, then press your elbows back against the inner thighs. Stay, then slowly come up, gently shake your hands and legs, and relax.

press the elbows backward

hold the ankles firmly

ARTICULATING NECK STRETCH

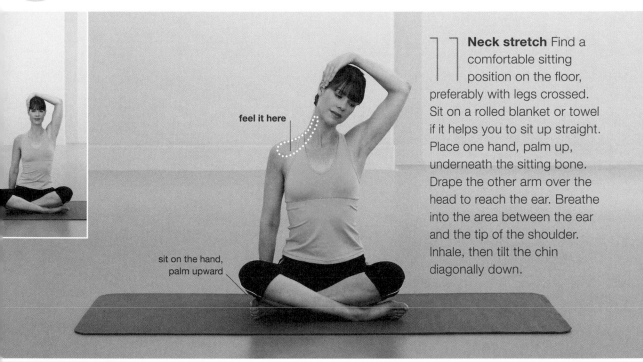

feel it here

sit on the hand,
palm upward

11 **Neck stretch** Find a comfortable sitting position on the floor, preferably with legs crossed. Sit on a rolled blanket or towel if it helps you to sit up straight. Place one hand, palm up, underneath the sitting bone. Drape the other arm over the head to reach the ear. Breathe into the area between the ear and the tip of the shoulder. Inhale, then tilt the chin diagonally down.

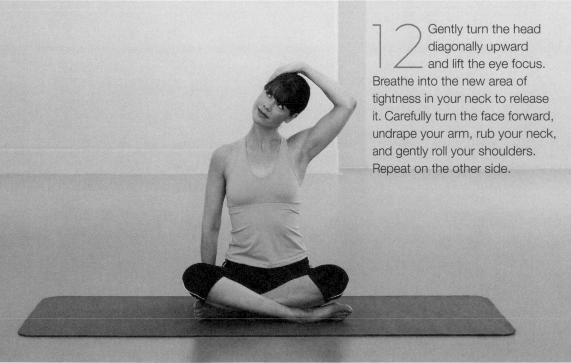

12 Gently turn the head diagonally upward and lift the eye focus. Breathe into the new area of tightness in your neck to release it. Carefully turn the face forward, undrape your arm, rub your neck, and gently roll your shoulders. Repeat on the other side.

ELONGATING KNEELING CAT

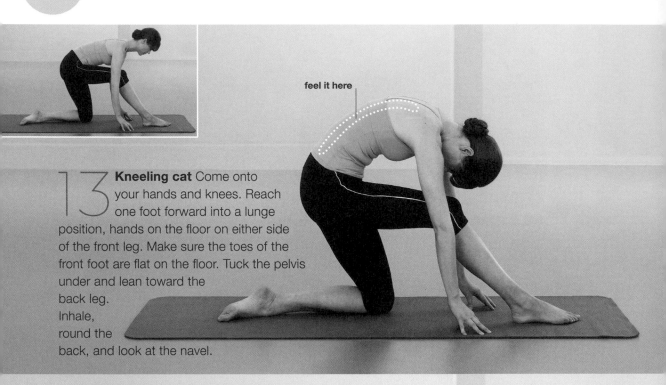

feel it here

13 **Kneeling cat** Come onto your hands and knees. Reach one foot forward into a lunge position, hands on the floor on either side of the front leg. Make sure the toes of the front foot are flat on the floor. Tuck the pelvis under and lean toward the back leg. Inhale, round the back, and look at the navel.

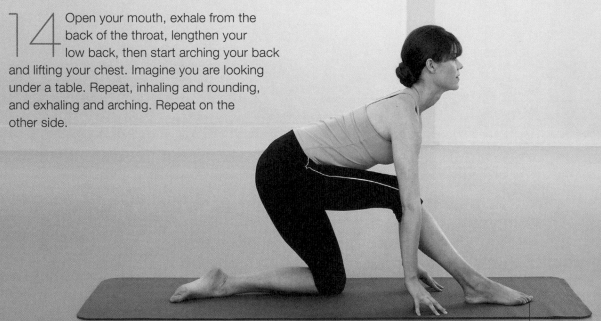

14 Open your mouth, exhale from the back of the throat, lengthen your low back, then start arching your back and lifting your chest. Imagine you are looking under a table. Repeat, inhaling and rounding, and exhaling and arching. Repeat on the other side.

toes stay down

BALANCING KNEELING SIDE STRETCH

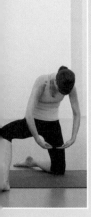

15 **Kneeling side stretch**
Starting on your hands and knees, take one leg diagonally in front, knee bent, sole of the foot on the floor. Turn both legs out slightly, lower the head, and take the arms in front of you, touching your middle fingers together. Then roll up through the spine and fan your arms open sideways.

16 Tuck your pelvis under and reach your top arm up and over toward the bent leg. Rest your lower forearm on the thigh of the bent leg. Reach up and out through the third finger of the top arm. Lift the groin muscles toward the head. Stay for 3 breath cycles, then repeat on the other side.

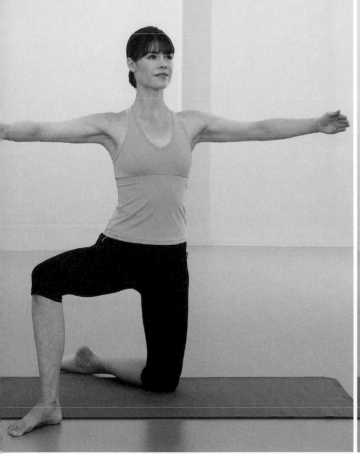

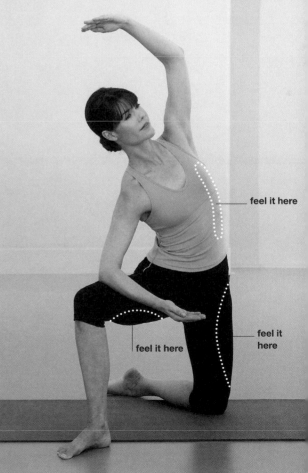

feel it here

feel it here

feel it here

CENTERING FISH STRETCH

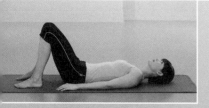

17 **Fish stretch** Lie on your back, knees bent, soles of the feet on the floor. Place your palms on the floor by your hips. Exhale, then gently press the low back forward and arch your back slightly.

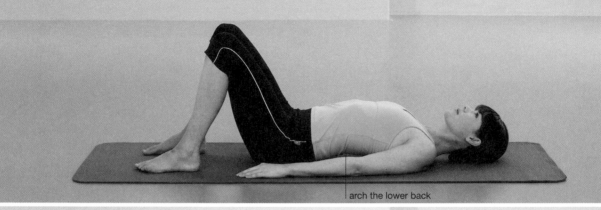

arch the lower back

18 Roll your shoulder blades back and down, then press down on your forearms and arch your back more to come up onto the top of your head. Put as little pressure on the head as possible. Stay for 1 long breath cycle. Relax, then repeat.

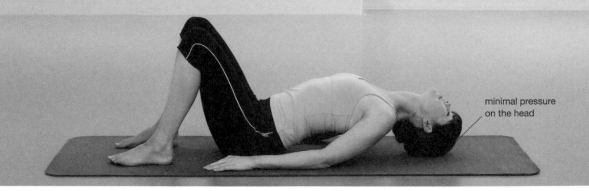

minimal pressure on the head

POWERING THIGH LUNGE

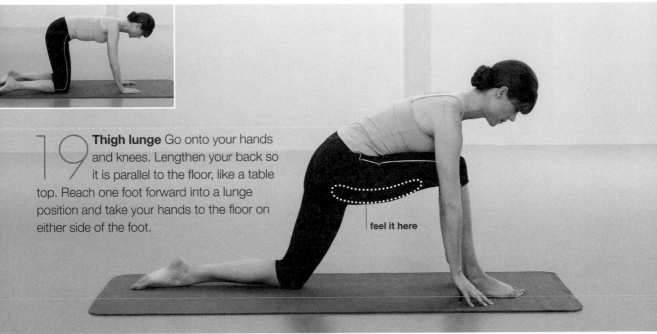

19 **Thigh lunge** Go onto your hands and knees. Lengthen your back so it is parallel to the floor, like a table top. Reach one foot forward into a lunge position and take your hands to the floor on either side of the foot.

feel it here

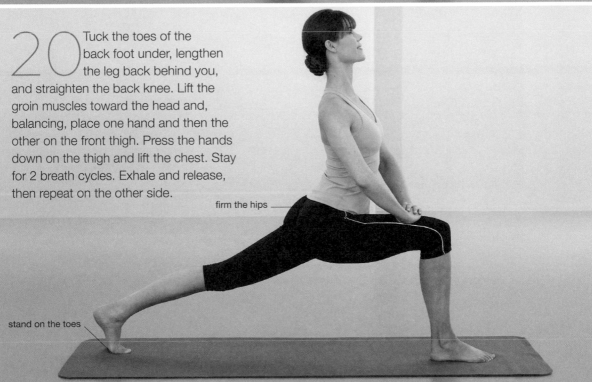

20 Tuck the toes of the back foot under, lengthen the leg back behind you, and straighten the back knee. Lift the groin muscles toward the head and, balancing, place one hand and then the other on the front thigh. Press the hands down on the thigh and lift the chest. Stay for 2 breath cycles. Exhale and release, then repeat on the other side.

firm the hips

stand on the toes

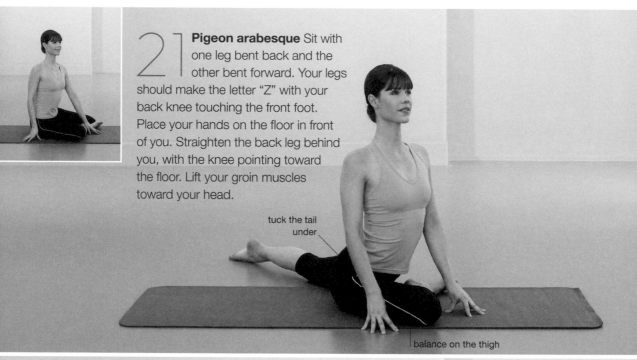

21 **Pigeon arabesque** Sit with one leg bent back and the other bent forward. Your legs should make the letter "Z" with your back knee touching the front foot. Place your hands on the floor in front of you. Straighten the back leg behind you, with the knee pointing toward the floor. Lift your groin muscles toward your head.

tuck the tail under

balance on the thigh

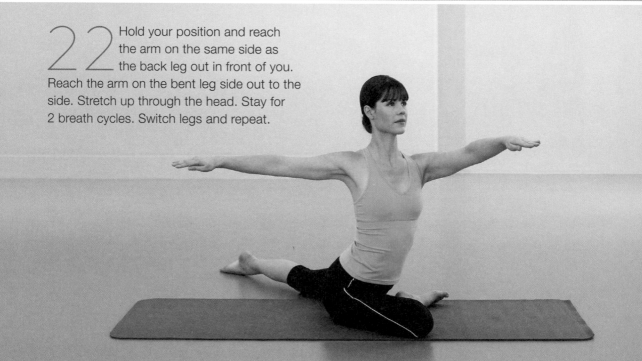

22 Hold your position and reach the arm on the same side as the back leg out in front of you. Reach the arm on the bent leg side out to the side. Stretch up through the head. Stay for 2 breath cycles. Switch legs and repeat.

ENERGIZING THE SPLIT

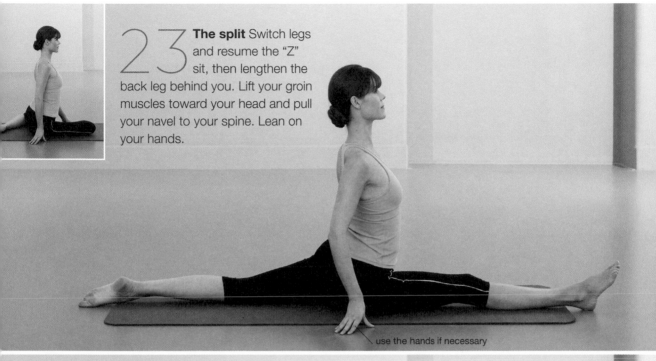

23 **The split** Switch legs and resume the "Z" sit, then lengthen the back leg behind you. Lift your groin muscles toward your head and pull your navel to your spine. Lean on your hands.

use the hands if necessary

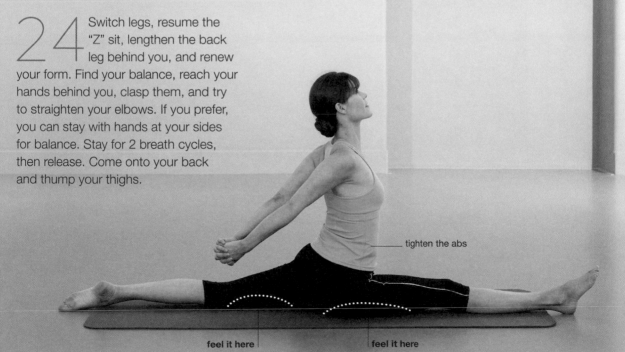

24 Switch legs, resume the "Z" sit, lengthen the back leg behind you, and renew your form. Find your balance, reach your hands behind you, clasp them, and try to straighten your elbows. If you prefer, you can stay with hands at your sides for balance. Stay for 2 breath cycles, then release. Come onto your back and thump your thighs.

tighten the abs

feel it here   feel it here

STRENGTH STRETCH AT A GLANCE

> LIMBERING BUTTERFLY STRETCH

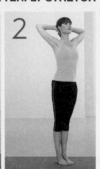

1

Page 82

2

Page 82

> OPENING UPPER SIDE BEND

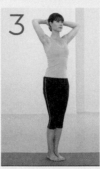

3

Page 83

4

Page 83

> LENGTHENING FLAT BACK SQUAT

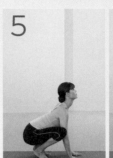

5

Page 84

6

Page 84

> ARTICULATING NECK STRETCH

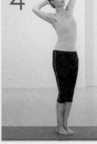

11

Page 87

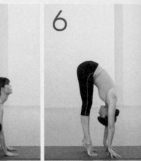

12

Page 87

> BALANCING KNEELING SIDE STRETCH

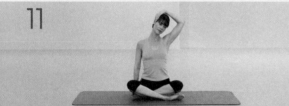

15

Page 89

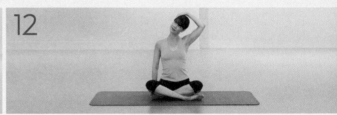

16

Page 89

> POWERING THIGH LUNGE

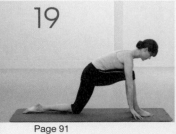

19

Page 91

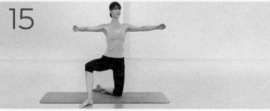

20

Page 91

> COORDINATING PIGEON ARABESQUE

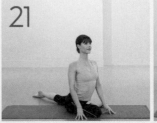

21

Page 92

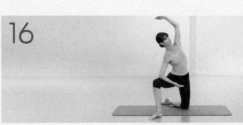

22

Page 92

> **STIMULATING WIDE SQUAT TWIST**

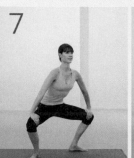

7

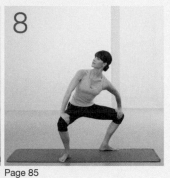

8

Page 85

Page 85

> **SUSTAINING DEEP SQUAT**

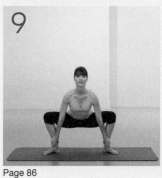

9

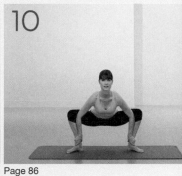

10

Page 86

Page 86

> **ELONGATING KNEELING CAT**

13

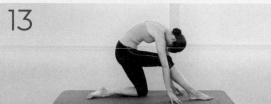

Page 88

14

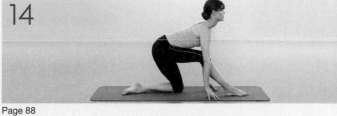

Page 88

> **CENTERING FISH STRETCH**

17

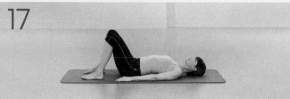
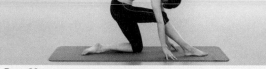

Page 90

18

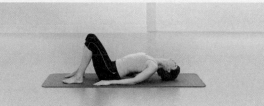

Page 90

> **ENERGIZING THE SPLIT**

23

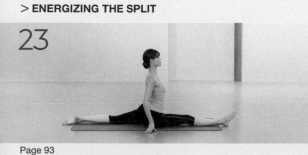

Page 93

24

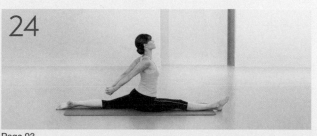

Page 93

STRENGTH STRETCH FAQS

Honesty and attention to detail are what make all the difference when it comes to bringing true strength to your stretch. Physical development takes time, so be patient. Here are some common questions and answers to help you in your quest to find your true physical potential.

I GET DIZZY DURING THE FLAT BACK SQUAT. IS THERE ANYTHING I CAN DO TO PREVENT THE DIZZINESS?

Dizziness is common when people first start doing upside-down exercises. The inner ear may not be used to inverting the head, and this is why you may feel some dizziness. But it's healthy to move the head in different orientations in an active movement for a limited time. The eyes usually control most of our balance. Simply keeping your eyes open and going slowly will help your body to acclimate to the position.

WHAT IF MY HIPS DON'T GO DOWN VERY FAR IN THE WIDE SQUAT TWIST AND THE DEEP SQUAT?

Just go down as far as you feel you can support the position. You'll still get a great groin stretch. Another option would be to hold onto a chair or other piece of furniture to steady yourself. Then you might find that you are able to bend more deeply into the squats. Consistent practice definitely makes for improvement in this stretch.

MY HEAD DOESN'T BEND WELL TO THE SIDE FOR THE NECK STRETCH. SHOULD I PULL HARDER?

First of all, never pull on the head; let gravity and the simple weight of the arm do the work. Over time it will open up. This is an exercise that truly requires precision and care in its execution. It gives a fabulous stretch of the different muscles of the neck. To access all those muscles, be sure to keep the head bent to the side, however slightly, as you turn your face.

I'M NOT FEELING MUCH STRETCH IN THE KNEELING CAT. HOW CAN I FIND THE STRETCH?

A common mistake here is to let the weight of the hip move toward the front leg. Be sure to keep the hips moving backward, especially as you lift the chest upward. Another tip is to literally stick your buttocks back and up, trying to arch the low back as you lift your chest. Yet another tip is to keep your chest as low as possible to the leg throughout the exercise.

I FEEL AS IF I'M NOT GOING ANYWHERE IN THE FISH STRETCH. IS THERE SOME TRICK TO IT?

Some people's body types mean they are able to arch their low back better than other people. It's purely structural. Don't ever force a position. If you can't get the stretch in this area, try propping a firm pillow or ball in between your shoulder blades. Practice by placing it there, bracing yourself onto your forearms, and squeezing between the shoulder blades for several breaths.

IS GOING INTO THE SPLIT NECESSARY TO CONSIDER MYSELF REALLY FLEXIBLE?

Not really. As with the Fish Stretch, body type often determines how naturally flexible you are. The main goal is a comfortable, pain-free body. Sometimes flexibility is undesirable, especially if a person's level of strength is too low to sustain the increased range of motion. A lithe body is preferable to a loose, disorganized body. That's why it's so important to emphasize the strength aspect as you develop your stretch.

HOW CAN THERE BE BOTH STRETCH AND STRENGTH IN ONE EXERCISE?

Strength is found in stretches by tensing the muscles in noncollapsed positions. Inversions and bending the spine over closed legs use your body weight as resistance to aid strengthening. Different bodily orientations, and moving hard-to-reach areas such as the rib cage create comprehensive strength. Strengthening many small parts leads to greater strength overall.

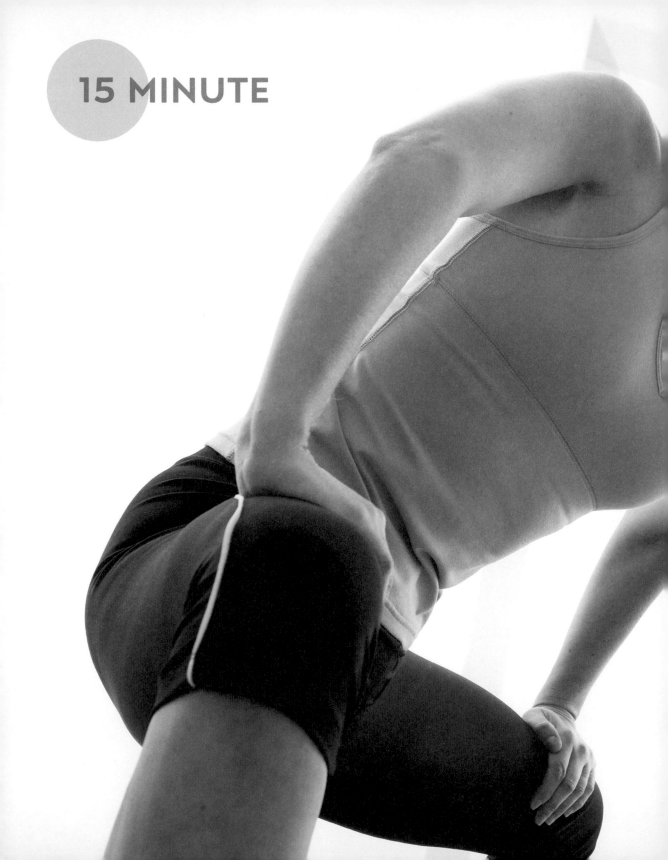

15 MINUTE

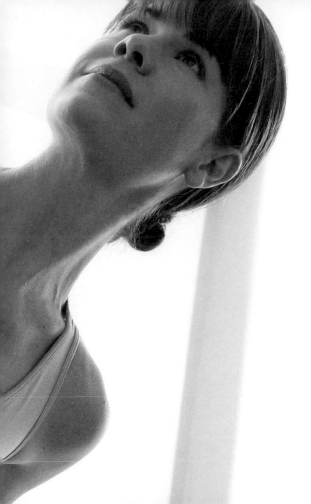

MOVING ON

LIFE PROPELS US INTO FORWARD MOTION
INCORPORATE STRETCHING FOR A HEALTHY LIFE

MODIFY AS NEEDED

It's not a failing to change an exercise to suit your needs, whether it's because of pain, age, or stiffness. There's a back door to every stretch. Nor is it cheating to use props and modifications. It's just plain wise.

The body can move in multiple directions with a great deal of ease, yet people are often deterred from doing stretching exercises because they worry about feeling discouraged. We would all love to look like the models featured in this book, but use them to help you see the stretching exercises clearly, not to compare yourself with them.

Some of the stretches may feel a little strange or unusual, especially if you are new to exercise. Part of the reason we stretch in unusual positions is to identify our weak links, so pay attention and focus on what feels too tight, too loose, or painful.

If an exercise doesn't feel right, there's always a way to make it more accessible. Some people have trouble sitting on the floor because they have tight hamstrings, glutes, or tightness in the low back, or a combination of one or more of these. Sitting on a footstool, ottoman, towel, or bolster can give just the lift needed to make the stretch possible.

Knees should never hurt during stretching. If they feel painful, support them on pillows or bolsters to take the pressure off. Another tip for this pose is to move the feet farther away from the groin.

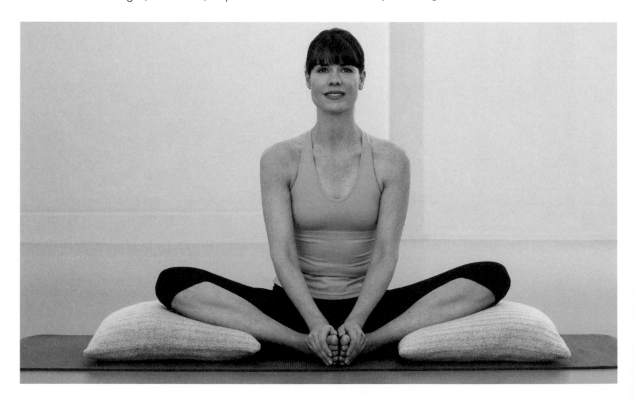

Pay special attention to your knees and monitor them for signs of pain or discomfort. "No pain, no gain" definitely does not apply to these complex joints. If you need to, prop them up with pillows when you are sitting to take the strain off the ligaments. If they feel tender when you kneel on them in weight-bearing positions, support them with some form of padding. Straighten them out of a bent-leg position if it's uncomfortable. If one of the knees refuses to straighten, as it might in the Lying Hamstring Stretch (see p69), use a towel, belt, or strap to reach the foot.

You can increase or decrease the intensity of a stretch as it suits you (perhaps your body feels different on different days or at different times of day) by pulling or extending more or less. Breathing and relaxing help you stretch farther. Alternatively, try modulating the intensity of a stretch by elongating in a progression from one to ten, and then reducing it. The level of intensity should never go into the "strain zone" and you should not have extreme pain after you have performed your stretches. Remember: compare only yourself to yourself to make the greatest gain.

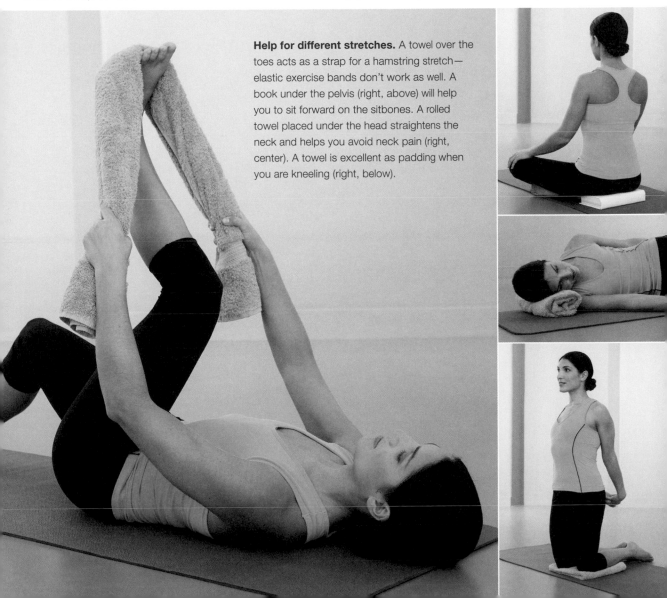

Help for different stretches. A towel over the toes acts as a strap for a hamstring stretch—elastic exercise bands don't work as well. A book under the pelvis (right, above) will help you to sit forward on the sitbones. A rolled towel placed under the head straightens the neck and helps you avoid neck pain (right, center). A towel is excellent as padding when you are kneeling (right, below).

STRETCHES FOR EVERYDAY LIFE

It's easy to take your stretches into everyday life. Notice how you move when you are grooming, dressing, even cooking and cleaning, and turn each movement into a stretch. And think "office" as well as "home" to get the most out of your stretch regimen.

Look at the ways your body moves in everyday life. Notice how different movements feel, such as brushing your hair or pulling on a sweater or pants. Does the task feel comfortable? Do you have the same range of motion from one side to another? How does it feel to bend over to reach to a pet? Let your answers to these questions guide you to set yourself goals that will make an action a little easier or smoother.

GRADUAL CHANGES
Changes to the way we move happen gradually over time. Diminishing range of motion creeps up on people of every age. A student notices writing arm and shoulders tightening during a long exam. A young mother notices a tight chest or sore low

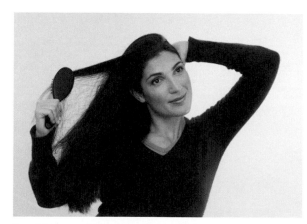

Brushing your hair is a great way to stretch the shoulders and chest. Try switching the brush to your nondominant hand to balance each side of the body.

back as she holds or reaches down to a toddler. Older adults notice they can't bend to the floor or reach up into cupboards as easily as in times past.

YOUR ADAPTABLE BODY
Life's distractions, such as being preoccupied with a demanding job, with a new baby, or with having to juggle a long commute with household duties can sideline us from regular physical activity. Then suddenly we notice a change and start to worry that our bodies are not as mobile as they once were.

The good news is that your body is adaptable. It changes to accept what the environment is telling it to do. If you inadvertently restrict its motions—for instance, by sitting for long periods—it adapts to the smaller, less frequent motions. Conversely, it can re-adapt. That's why it's important to find ways in everyday life to get an extra little bit of stretch. Small changes can keep your body healthy over time.

IN A CROWDED SCHEDULE
It's commendable to devote an hour or two a day to getting exercise, but not everyone can do that. Our 15-minute programs make it possible to get exercise, even with the most crowded schedule. Yet neither should you overlook the power of taking 25 seconds—four breath cycles—to feel the stretch in an everyday position or movement. This will add to your overall physical well-being. Using this strategy during those overwhelming times of life, when every second appears to be accountable, will pay off handsomely.

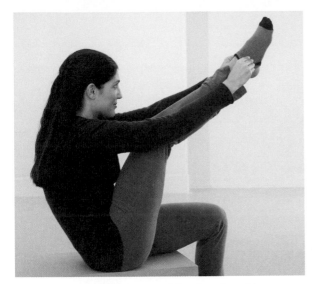

Putting on your socks is a good time for a hamstring stretch. Simply lift the leg, or reach over to it, bow the head, and take a few breaths.

Working in an office gives you a good opportunity to use some chair stretches from the Wake Up The Stretch program (see pp26–29). Reach your hands behind your head and wing your elbows open in a chest stretch. It helps your workday go faster and more smoothly. Sitting work is probably some of the most tiring, and it's important to take frequent breaks, even for a few breaths. Office stretches increase clear thinking as well as helping to avoid computer overuse problems that can affect your chest, hands, and arms. Intermittent breathing and stretches will make you a more productive worker, whatever you do for a living.

AN EVERYDAY HABIT

Perseverance is simple when you make stretches an everyday habit. Habits can be formed in as little as 21 days, so set a goal on your calendar for the next 21 days and find opportunities for a stretch at home, work, and play. Have faith: the body will change, but only with persistence. Stretching in everyday life makes that persistence easy.

Take a twist break at the office. Cross one leg over the other and turn in the direction of the crossed leg, just as in our Seated Cross-leg Twist (see p28).

EVERYDAY STRETCHES THAT MAKE A DIFFERENCE

- **Reach a little farther** to stretch into that pantry. Take a break. Yawn to stretch the jaw. Open the eyes and look upward to open the chest and neck.

- **Stretch your legs and hips** when putting on and taking off clothes. Practice lunges when vacuuming and move your hips from side to side when sweeping.

- **Renew your posture at the office** by squeezing between the shoulder blades and rolling your shoulders. Firm the glutes and sit up tall.

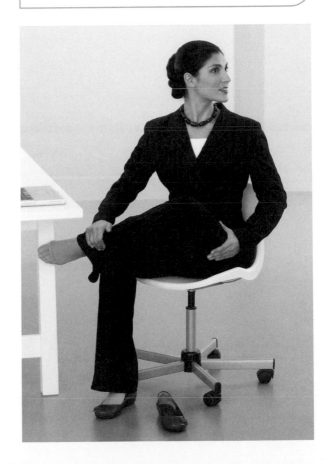

RELAXATION TECHNIQUES

Relaxation takes discipline in a busy world. Chores, obligations, and crises sap energy reserves and present roadblocks to emotional balance. Try these scheduled and unscheduled calming techniques to make relaxation a priority in your life.

Relaxation is great for renewing the body, mind, and spirit. During every waking hour we expend our physical and mental energy, so we need to replenish it. Take a cue from professional athletes who aim for peak fitness. They know that the key to achieving optimal functioning lies in alternating periods of stress with times of relief and rest.

We all need a certain amount of stress in our lives to challenge and motivate us. But we also need to shake off any fatigue on a regular basis to avoid chronic weariness.

SLEEP AND REST

It's important for us all to renew our resources with nightly sleep and timely rest. Developing a healthy nightly ritual is essential in establishing an optimal renewal plan. Make your bedroom a sanctuary by creating a soothing, quiet place with your favorite

Use the contract–release method to lessen the tensions in your body. One by one, tighten and release each body part. End by tensing your whole body (inset, below), then let go and breathe deeply (main picture, below).

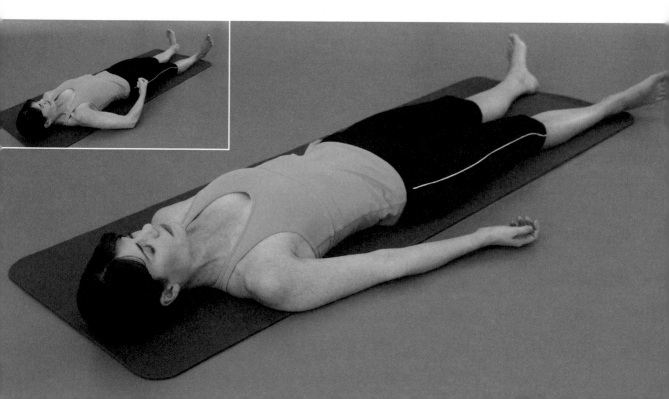

TIPS FOR DEALING WITH DAILY STRESS

- **To cope with life's ups and downs** be sure to make time daily for refreshment and restoration.

- **Manage your stress.** Try a progressive relaxation technique, breathe deeply, or learn to meditate to reverse the effects of stress.

- **Develop good sleep hygiene.** Make your bedroom an inviting, quiet, peaceful sanctuary and let go of the day's hassles and worries.

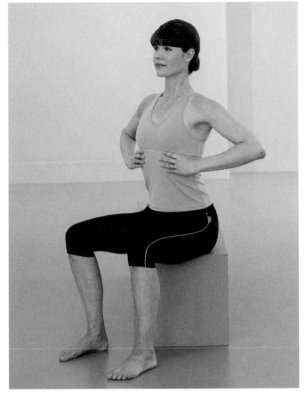

Practice deep breathing. The diaphragmatic breath is found by placing your fingers at the bottom of your breast bone and sniffing or coughing a few times. Inhale deeply; feel the rib cage expand.

bedding and gentle lighting. Don't have the television or your computer in the bedroom. It should be a space strictly for unwinding.

Don't drink alcohol last thing at night. Instead, savor a cup of a caffeine-free drink for an uninterrupted night's slumber. Some people find a warm bath before bed helps to relax them. Light reading material can also quiet the mind and help you leave the day's worries behind you. Make sure the room is completely dark while you're asleep. Studies have shown that exposure to light during sleep can disturb your body's natural cycles.

If you awaken during the night, focus on the pleasant texture of the bedding, take deep breaths, and relish the luxurious time you have for rest. Strive to get seven to eight hours of the deep sleep you need for complete physical restoration.

USING STRETCHING TO HELP YOU RELAX

Relaxation techniques can greatly influence the restoration cycle. Simple exercises such as the progressive contract–relax technique (see opposite) can quickly lower body tension and take your mind away from overly analytical thoughts. For instance, tense the fists as you count to ten, then relax them. In order of progression, apply the same tense-then-

relax method to the shoulders, thighs, calves, feet, abdomen, and finally the face, puckering your lips and eyes strongly. End the technique by tensing your entire body, and then completely let go of all your body tension as you breathe five deep, long breaths. Notice how relaxed your body and your mind have become.

Another simple yet reliable relaxation technique, excellent for any setting and any location, is deep diaphragmatic breathing (see above). Place your fingers at the bottom of your breastbone to find the way your diaphragm moves. Sniff quickly several times or cough to feel the muscles move. Breathe into the diaphragm and feel these muscles expand for four seconds (think "1-alligator, 2-alligator", etc.). Then exhale for 8 seconds. Slow breathing reverses the fight-or-flight, adrenaline-based panic that's part of our fast-paced society.

STRATEGIES FOR HEALTHY LIVING

We all strive to achieve a good quality of life, whether we're just starting out or have reached retirement. Work, play, good nutrition, and the ability to relish the joys and cope with the disappointments of life are all a part of the equation that will bring us health and contentment.

Wouldn't you rather live in a high-functioning, optimal way than a low-functioning one? Physically, we need energy to meet the demands of the day. We want to move around and lift and bend without pain or limitation, which is where the stretching programs in this book come into play. Mentally, we want to be alert and keep our homes and jobs running well. Emotionally, it is preferable to be stable, acting instead of reacting, in our family and professional encounters.

BALANCE AND POSITIVITY

There are many things in life that we cannot control, so focus on those you can. A good starting point is a healthy, well-balanced diet. Eat five servings of fruits and vegetables and about three 3-ounce servings of protein (meat, fish, dairy, eggs, grains, legumes, nuts) per day. Also limit your intake of starches (potatoes and bread) and fats (butter and oils). Doctors recommend that we eat six small meals a day. This ignites the metabolism, provides brain food, and promotes a steady emotional state.

Another key is to balance your activities between work and play. Work may be essential for a living, but don't make it your life. Take up a hobby. Walk outdoors; breathe deeply. Even developing a sense of humor adds play into the day. Nurture your rest and sleep habits (see p104). Relaxation techniques, meditation, and good, sound sleep are building blocks that add to the foundation of health.

Finally, never forget that you choose your attitude. A positive attitude rises to the challenge

ADDING QUALITY TO YOUR LIFE

- **Be proactive** in balancing healthy nutrition, activity, and rest.
- **Select fresh seasonal foods.** Divide your plate in two. Fill one half of it with fruits or vegetables. Then split the other half between a protein and a serving of starch.
- **Balance work with play.** Find a hobby and your funny bone. Cherish family and friends. Get outdoors. Take time to rest and recharge.
- **Protect and nurture** a positive outlook. See how it helps you deal with life's challenges and "failed experiments."

of discouragement and changing circumstances, Aggressively preserve your positive outlook; seek out positive people. And acknowledge the big picture of life, with its cycle of peaks and valleys.

The perfect hobby presents a challenge and gives an opportunity for mastery outside your regular routine. Taking your stretching to another level, perhaps by joining a yoga class, will challenge you to go further and find your inner grace and balance. You might be surprised by what you achieve when you "go for it."

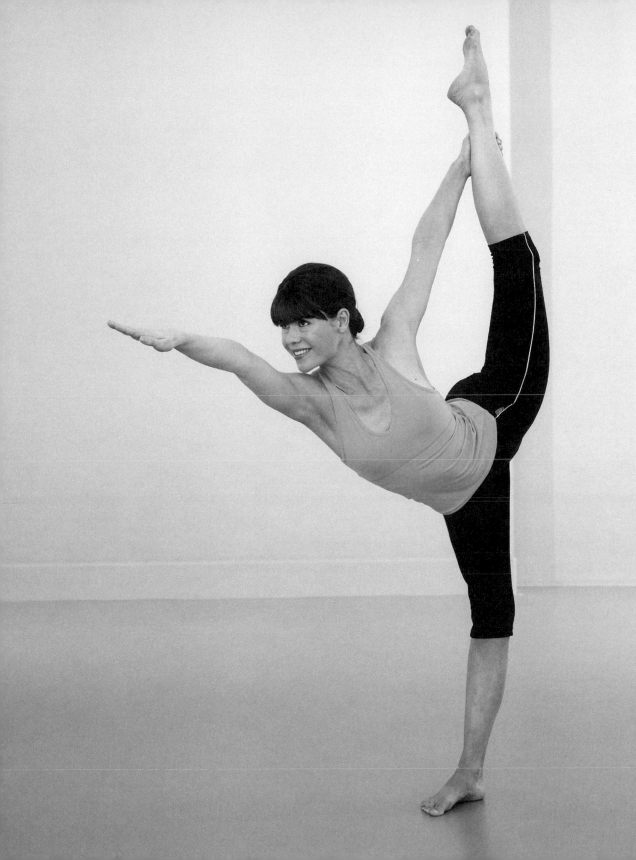

USEFUL RESOURCES

Taking a proactive stance toward your health care will pay off royally.
A comprehensive program of health care entails first getting your
own team of health-care practitioners together, as well as organizing
your own health-care strategy for healthy living.

Stretching comes under several categories and can be integrated into other programs such as fitness, Pilates, physiotherapy, yoga, and dance. Here are some resources to get you started.

FITNESS

The American Council on Exercise

www.acefitness.org
ACE is a nonprofit organization committed to enriching quality of life through safe and effective physical activity. ACE protects all segments of society against ineffective fitness products, programs, and trends through its ongoing public education, outreach, and research. ACE further protects the public by setting certification and continuing education standards for fitness professionals.

The American College of Sports Medicine

www.acsm.org
ACSM promotes and integrates scientific research, education, and practical applications of sports medicine and exercise science to maintain and enhance physical performance, fitness, health, and quality of life.

PILATES

Pilates Method Alliance

pilatesmethodalliance.org
The Pilates Method Alliance (PMA) is the international not-for-profit professional association for the Pilates method. The PMA's mission is to protect the public by establishing certification and continuing education standards for Pilates professionals.

YOGA

Iyengar Yoga Association

iyengar-yoga.com
The Iyengar method of yoga is initially learned through the in-depth study of asanas (posture) and pranayama (breath control). Mr. Iyengar has systematized over 200 classical yoga asanas and 14 different types of pranayamas. These have been structured and categorized so as to allow a beginner to progress surely and safely from basic postures to the most advanced as they gain flexibility, strength, and sensitivity in mind, body, and spirit.

Ashtanga Yoga Institute

kpjayshala.com
Ashtanga Yoga is an ancient system of yoga that was taught by Vamana Rishi in the *Yoga Korunta*. This text was imparted to Sri T. Krishnamacharya in the early 1900s by his guru Rama Mohan Brahmachari, and was later passed down to Pattabhi Jois.

Anusara Yoga

anusarayoga.com
Anusara (a-nu-sar-a), means "flowing with grace," "going with the flow," "following your heart." Founded by John Friend in 1997, Anusara Yoga is a powerful hatha yoga system that unifies a Tantric philosophy of Intrinsic Goodness with Universal Principles of Alignment™.

PHYSICAL THERAPY

The American Physical Therapy Association

www.apta.org
The mission of the American Physical Therapy Association (APTA), the principal membership organization representing and promoting the profession of physical therapy, is to further the profession's role in the prevention, diagnosis, and treatment of movement dysfunctions and the enhancement of the physical health and functional abilities of members of the public.

PEDRO (Physiotherapy Evidence Database)

An online database of randomized controlled trials and systematic reviews in physiotherapy. It can be accessed free of charge at: www.pedro.fhs.usyd.edu.au/

NUTRITION

nutridiary.com
This free online food and exercise diary will help you analyze and chart your diet and activity level so that you can attain your diet goals. Whether you want to maintain, lose, or gain weight, having a goal and keeping track is a great motivator to stick with a healthy eating and exercise program.

DVDS BY SUZANNE MARTIN

The following useful DVDs are available to purchase at pilatestherapeutics.com/shop.

Pilates Therapeutics® The Upper Core: Exercises for a Pain-Free Life (2002)
This DVD was developed to respond to the prevalence of repetitive stress injuries of the shoulders, arms, and hands.

Pilates Therapeutics® The Pelvic Core: More Exercise for a Pain-Free Life (2002)
This DVD focuses on 24 balancing exercises to help low back and pelvic pain, knee problems, and post-pregnancy restoration.

Pilates Therapeutics® The Scoliosis Management Series

Scoliosis Series Part 1: Management & Improvement featuring Wall Springs (2006)
Part 1 is designed to help persons who have scoliosis, or abnormal curvature of the spine.

Scoliosis Series Part 2: Breathing Exercises as Part of Scoliosis Management (2007)
Part 2 continues the concepts for managing scoliosis from Part 1, but focuses on breathing for long-term management.

Pilates Therapeutics® A Step-Wise Approach to Post-Natal Restoration (2007)
This DVD is designed to be of use to anyone who has given birth in the last 18 months or will give birth.

Pilates Therapeutics® Breast Cancer Survivor's Guide to Physical Restoration (2007)
This DVD is for those who have had or will have surgeries related to breast cancer treatment.

To contact Suzanne Martin
pilatestherapeutics.com

INDEX

ACKNOWLEDGMENTS

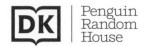

Penguin Random House

ABOUT SUZANNE MARTIN

Suzanne is a doctor of physical therapy, an exercise physiologist, and a gold-certified Pilates expert. A former dancer, she is a Master trainer certified by the American Council on Exercise. She is published by *Dance Magazine,* Dorling Kindersley, and the *Journal of Dance Medicine and Science,* among others. She is also well known as an educator on Pilates, dance, and physical therapy. Suzanne has been the lead physical therapist for the Smuin Ballet in San Francisco for more than 20 years and maintains a private practice in Marietta, Georgia. For more information, check her website: www.pilatestherapeutics.com.

From the first edition
AUTHOR'S ACKNOWLEDGMENTS

So many thanks to all my teachers, mentors, clients, and students who challenged me to break a movement down into its essence so that I can now pass it on to you. Thanks to my scoliosis and injuries that forced me to find ways to help myself and then to help others. Thanks to DK for being willing to include many concepts and unusual images in this book and to communicate them around the world. A special thanks to Hilary Mandleberg, Jenny Latham, Mary-Clare Jerram, Miranda Fenton, Helen McTeer, Ruth Jenkinson, and Anne Fisher and Susan Downing for their patience, and for working so hard to help me realize my dreams.

PUBLISHER'S ACKNOWLEDGMENTS

Dorling Kindersley thanks photographer Ruth Jenkinson and her assistant Carly Churchill; Viv Riley at Touch Studios; the models Sam Magee and Tara Lee; Rachel Jones for the hair and makeup; Sweaty Betty for the loan of exercise clothing; Peter Kirkham for proofreading, and Hilary Bird for the index. For design assistance on the second edition: Saumya Agarwal and Rajdeep Singh.

SECOND EDITION
US Editor Lori Hand
Editor Megan Lea
Designer Tessa Bindloss
DTP Designers Satish Chandra Gaur, Umesh Singh Rawat
Senior DTP Designer Tarun Sharma
Jacket Designer Amy Cox
Jacket Coordinator Lucy Philpott
Senior Production Editor Tony Phipps
Senior Production Controller Luca Bazzoli
Managing Editor Ruth O'Rourke
Managing Art Editor Marianne Markham
Art Director Maxine Pedliham
Publishing Director Katie Cowan

FIRST EDITION
Project Editor Hilary Mandleberg
Senior Editor Jennifer Latham
Managing Editor Dawn Henderson
Art Director Peter Luff
Stills Photography Ruth Jenkinson
US Editor Jenny Siklós
Project Art Editor Helen McTeer
Senior Art Editor Susan Downing
Managing Art Editor Christine Keilty
Publisher Mary-Clare Jerram

Video produced for Dorling Kindersley by
Chrome Productions www.chromeproductions.com
Director Robin Schmidt
DOP Marcus Domleo, Matthew Cooke
Camera Joe McNally, Marcus Domleo, Jonathan Iles
Production Manager Hannah Chandler
Production Assistant Azra Gul
Grip Pete Nash
Gaffer Paul Wilcox, Johann Cruickshank
Music Chad Hobson
Hair and Make-up Victoria Barnes
Voiceover Suzanne Pirret
Voiceover Recording Ben Jones

This American Edition, 2022
First American Edition, 2010
Published in the United States by DK Publishing
1450 Broadway, Suite 801, New York, NY 10018

A catalog record for this book is available from the Library of Congress
ISBN 978-0-7440-5129-2

DK books are available at special discounts when purchased in bulk for sales promotions, premiums, fund-raising, or educational use. For details, contact: DK Publishing Special Markets, 1450 Broadway, Suite 801, New York, New York 10018 or SpecialSales@dk.com

Printed and bound in China.

For the curious
www.dk.com

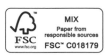

MIX
Paper from responsible sources
FSC™ C018179

This book was made with Forest Stewardship Council ™ certified paper—one small step in DK's commitment to a sustainable future. For more information, go to www.dk.com/our-green-pledge